"During the time my wif suring gift to be able to call our friend Rob Lane, noted oncologist. With his extensive medical background and expertise, he was able to compassionately guide us step-by-step through the maze of questions and concerns. So much of what he taught us has gone into the book and blog, *The Bell Lap*, and is why Joni and I heartily recommend it. It's a tremendous no-nonsense guide for anyone battling cancer. In a way it could be considered as part of a cancer-warrior's support group. It is like having an instant "2nd opinion" from a skilled medical oncologist – one who knows how to dispense complex information in a sensible and compassionate way. Joni and I agree that this book is needed. It should be published."

-Ken Tada and Joni Eareckson Tada, Authors, Patient

"I just read the first 3 chapters of your book and think it's great! I think chapters 1 and 2 will save/preserve my sanity. I have a friend who is being treated for PTSD and anxiety/depression 8 years after her successful colon cancer treatment – these chapters could have saved her an endless amount of anguish!"

-Jana Heyd, Attorney, Patient

"Never in my career have I encountered such a useful book – and I've looked. The pearls of wisdom you have strung together apply to all of us. It's a wonderful roadmap for defeating the

Dragon in our lives, whether summoned by cancer or by another demon. As a nurse in a critical care unit most of my life, I was always an advocate for my critical patients but could have done that much better if *The Bell Lap* had been available to me then.

-**Alice Markowitz, RN**, Critical Care Nurse, Patient

"If you've been diagnosed with cancer, you know the pit in your stomach and the lump in your throat. This book will put the hope back in your heart and help you regain the control of your life!"

-**Lisa Bjerke**, Patient

"I am just about to finish your book. It is been extremely insightful and just what I needed to read at this time. I hope to be able to convey the information to my brother without being pedantic and making sure that his decisions and feelings are on the forefront."

-**Amy**, Sister of a patient

"This is the book I wish I had available during the course of my cancer diagnosis and treatment. It answers so many of those questions that we often don't even know to ask! Even though the book wasn't available, at least the author was."

-**Sue Wright**, Patient

"Walking alongside people who have just found out that their test results are positive and a cancer must be treated is an earth-shaking experience. The uncertainty of that moment with the anxiety they feel and the fear of death in the forefront of their minds leaves them in a daze of confusion. Usually, as their pastor, they call me on their way home from the doctor's office looking for assurance that everything is going to be all right. Yet, unless you are a cancer survivor yourself responding is difficult. "The Bell Lap" by Dr. Lane provides pastors and caregivers a resource that allows us to travel this journey with people whose lives are impacted by cancer. It is written in a way that helps pastors understand the prognosis, grasp the treatments available, and provides the hope to sustain the people they serve in their churches.

-Gino Grunberg, Pastor

"When I received my cancer diagnosis at age 58, I was unprepared to say the least. I had never seriously considered this as a possibility and it's impossible to overstate how shocking, unsettling and disorienting that news was. It was like getting hit by a bolt of lightning. One minute life is normal and the next the tables have been overturned. If you or a loved one or friend is dealing with cancer, I strongly recommend reading "The Bell Lap." In this insightful book, Dr. Lane provides a clear and concise roadmap on how to recover one's equilibrium, how to engage the many questions and issues that cancer forces upon you, and how to live life fully even in the face of the devastating news."

-**Dave Bjerke,** Patient

"I commend you for your writing and care for those who will benefit from your years of experience. Gale and I certainly appreciate you tender counsel as we faced the unknown pathway before us. It's interesting that those 2 ½ to 3 years were some of the sweetest of our years together. There's so much to learn in the midst of the discomfort of such an illness. Thank you for your friendship."

-**David Williams**, husband of a Patient

CANCER'S BELL LAP

and THE DRAGON BEHIND THE DOOR

Strategies for Running the Bell Lap and Defeating the Dragon

CANCER
The Bell Has Rung
Might Be Your Last Lap?
Better Run as If It Is!
Outrace the Dragon
Stay the Course
FINISH STRONG

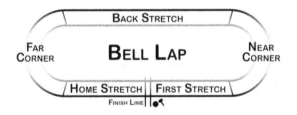

ROBERT LANE, M.D.
A Handbook for Seriously Engaging Cancer

Dedication

To Wendell W. Price, who opened our eyes to the richness
of purpose one's life can have in spite of cancer,
and how victory over leukemia or cancer is about
so much more than just staying alive.

And to the cancer patients of Northwest Cancer Center
and Puget Sound Cancer Centers whose courageous
lives now guide our decisions.

Acknowledgements

Many thanks to the team of patients, counselors, pastors, colleagues, nurses, and friends who have made this book possible: first to my enduring wife, Suzanne, whose counsel and encouragement have been essential, then to my special friend and cancer survivor, Sue Wright, who devoted hours to teaching me from her own experience and to proof reading the manuscript through grace-loving eyes, and to Mark Knowlden, Suzanne Kirsch, and Rick Enloe who labored through the roughest first draft and whose enthusiasm rescued it from the dust bin. Thanks also to Sandy Brannon, Debbie Gregory, Alice Markowitz, and Gino Grunberg for their insights and corrections.

Much gratitude to my editor, Dr. Larry Keefauver (www. ymcs.org) for honing my prose and the staff at Xulon Press for their energy and skill in bringing this project to fruition.

The talented Ty Knowlden (https://m.facebook.com/pro-file.php?) translated my metaphorical imagery of the dragon that haunts fearful people into riveting pictures for both the blog CancerDocTalk.Com and the book.

The web wizard, Jason Neighbors (www.JasonNeighbors. com) has been an entertaining and creative resource to guide my interaction with digital media and design my websites.

The creative Chris Ballasiotes (Ballasiotes Marketing/Media, Fox Island, WA) brought his skill as a storyteller and videographer to bear in creating visual vignettes of patient's lives as recounted in the book. They are now used on the blog CancerDocTalk.com as guiding adjuncts to the book.

Table of Contents

Introduction

Size Up the Competition, Meet the Enemy

Thirty years of caring for cancer patients has taught me you are fighting a war on two fronts—one conventional and the other unconventional. You are facing two adversaries, one you can see and one you can't. One of these adversaries you can feel and measure. It is called a malignancy that attacks your body. The other enemy you can only sense in the dark. I call it the "Dragon." It attacks your life, seductively at first, so you are only able to sense its trepidation.

Doctors go after the cancer cells invading your body with weapons you can at least somewhat understand, like surgery, radiation, and chemotherapy, but those don't work against the Dragon and with it you are on your own! You are on your own against it as it assaults your life in a guerilla-like warfare that is psychological and spiritual aimed at your emotions, mind, and spirit. The Dragon may not be able to kill you with guilt, doubt, fear, and anger, but it can disable you enough that you cannot fight the cancer in your body that wants to kill .

This book is different than most on cancer. It is going to show you how to wage war on both fronts. It will help you beat back the biologic malignancy and it is also going to flush out the Dragon, expose its weapons, beat back its onslaught on your life, and ultimately defeat it. Life after a cancer diagnosis plays out phase by phase, stage by stage, and season by season. It is a physical, psychological, and spiritual battle fought over months and years in ways that are hard to grasp at the outset, but essential to anticipate if your intent is to win the war.

A foot race on an oval track is a good metaphor for a life with cancer. In racing, the last lap is announced by the ringing of a bell. Too often in life, it is announced by the diagnosis of cancer or some other potentially fatal disease. In racing, the length of that last lap, the bell lap, is known, but in life it is not. However, in both a race and in life, the bell signals it is time for your best and perhaps final effort—at least that is the way it feels. In life, it might be shorter than you hope or expect, therefore, it deserves your best effort from the get-go.

The racetrack is divided into five segments: There is the *first stretch* which leads into the *near corner* then rounds into the *backstretch*. That leads to the *far corner* which breaks on to the *home stretch* that ends at the finish line. After a cancer diagnosis rings your bell, life will play out with similar phases. Each phase will have its own challenges and opportunities. Each segment deserves special attention and needs its own unique strategy.

This metaphorical race isn't about what is going on in your physical body that you seem to have little or no control over. It's about the repercussions of the disease in your life that are affected by your mind, emotions, and spirit which you can control. Like in a foot race, you will have competition along the way. The Dragon will come at you from a different direction in each track segment or phase of cancer life. It will be like a troll under the track, rising up to challenge you at any moment by whispering words of discouragement, confusion or defeat.

Cancer strikes boldly at your body, but the Dragon sneaks into your life unseen at first. Your attention will be focused with the doctors on how to defeat and destroy the cancer in your body. However, the Dragon can't be killed through medication; it will never leave your life, but it can be defeated. You cannot out run it until you recognize it, but you need a long range plan to outsmart and conquer it. Otherwise, it will haunt you in the same way PTSD haunts soldiers even after the battle is over and won. You must go after it methodically, like an athlete who prepares a plan for a race and sticks to it. Every competitor knows there will be a final lap which will be announced by a ringing bell. Their whole race is preparation for their finest effort in that final lap.

Cancer will ring that bell for many of us and announce that our bell lap has begun. However, unlike a foot race, there is no telling how long your final lap will last.

**Only a Dragon-defeating strategy
will make it a lap worth living and ensure victory.**

The Plan

We will talk about the challenges and how to overcome them, the opportunities and how to grab them, and about the Dragon and how to defeat it. In sports, we race to win. In a war, we fight to prevail. So, that is just how we approach life with cancer. With the gift of life at birth, we inherited the certainty of losing it and the uncertainty of knowing when. That is normal, but how we respond defines each of us and that is what really matters.

Grieving your potential loss is necessary and worthy of your attention. So don't be surprised by grief, but also don't be surprised when an undefeated dragon uses it to knock you off the track and disable you. Do not let that happen. Give grief the respect it deserves, perhaps some each day, but keep it in its place. Then step around it and live your precious life.

Come journey through the lives of my patients, and see if you can find in their stories some clues for your own bell lap. Perhaps, they will speak some of the same truths to you that they have spoken to me. I was surprised by how much there is to learn, as neither medical school nor life had prepared me for what they had to teach.

I have written a pair of books to share all that I have learned. This is the first, which focuses on cancer and is very practical, covering important things to consider either as a cancer patient, a family member or a caregiver. Most of it applies to anyone with any serious illness. There is always a Dragon behind the door and it is always snipping at us. Identifying it and keeping it at bay during treatment will be the focus of this book. Defeating it completely is deferred to the second book, *The Cancer Bell Lap Windrunners & the Dragon Vanquished*. This second book chronicles the lives of the *Windrunners*, those who run their bell laps, struggle, and even stumble, but run better, faster, and often longer than everyone else because they run in the right direction and with the wind. They are the ones who plot their course, lighten their load, smote the Dragon early, and then run expectantly, less impeded, like the wind, into their future.

Although both books seem to be addressed to cancer patients, they are applicable to anyone. Surely, not everyone will have cancer, but everyone will face death and meet the Dragon along the way if they haven't already. Cancer simply brings the Dragon out of hiding and into the light where we can deal with it *or* eventually die with it.

There are hosts of half comprehended, faulty notions that float around the minds of the afflicted. Often, those notions are allowed to take up residence unchallenged, only to haunt our quiet times and steal our joy. I want to flush out each one, so they can be cut down to size and overcome with truth. There is life *after* cancer. There is life *with* cancer, but we have to defeat the Dragon who would tell us otherwise to really experience it.

With the Dragon, come the existential questions we all must face one day. The day those questions are asked and answered will make every other day better, no matter how many or how few there are left. Most who hurdle those questions and land squarely on the track with answers, look back to thank whatever rang their bell or to pat themselves on the back for ringing their own bell.

While most wisdom is learned experientially the hard way, it is often easier to discover if you have seen what it looks like in a winner's life—someone like the Windrunners. If your bell has rung or even if it hasn't, I hope you can catch up with one of the Windrunners and see how it is done. First, though, hear the bell, get running, and identify the Dragon. You can do it because it is not about a physical performance, but about choices and decisions.

It is not about those things outside your control, but the ones squarely within your control.

The Starting Line

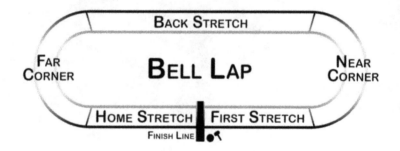

Chapter 1

On Your Mark, Get Set

The Starting Line

Suspense, mystery, and uncertainty! We love the excitement that each brings to our movies and sporting events, but not within our own lives. A horn announces the beginning of the fourth quarter of a football game, a buzzer heralds the last two minutes of a basketball game, and a bell sounds the last lap of a long distance foot track race. When cancer rings that bell in life uncertainty arrives, suspense builds, and dread covers it all. An ending is certain, but the outcome is unknown!

If cancer has announced your bell lap, what will you do? No one enters a race to lose, yet some in the *human* race collapse on the track when the bell rings, or they just turn tail and take off in the wrong direction. This book is not about them. It's about those who set out to win, not just in terms of health, but also in life.

Anyone can be victorious, but it doesn't come easily or without work. No one can do it for you. This is do-it-yourself stuff. You can't buy it. You can't hire it out. You are the only contestant in your race. Winning doesn't look the same for everyone, but it feels the same—triumphant, peaceful, and free!

To get on the winner's podium, you have to first hear the bell and acknowledge what it means. Then, you must deal decisively with the issues of the first stretch. It is essential that you identify and cope with the Dragon in the near corner and then shift into overdrive in the backstretch where you decide what really matters and what you will hope for during the rest of your race. Once you discover who you really are and what baggage you don't need, you can lighten your load, focus on your course, and joyfully run to make your life count. The far corner is for passing the baton and getting ready for your final power play down the home stretch.

Although I have met a number of patients who started running too late, I've never met anyone who started too hard or too soon. I do know many who have started to run hard and discovered the finish line often seemed to keep moving outward in front of them. It was because they didn't focus on the end, but how they were running.

Living in a newfound purpose has to become the focus.

When the word *cancer* rings the bell, the very ground shakes, vision blurs, and *everyone* stumbles. No one can quite see the finish line, but all of a sudden they become aware it is out there looming vaguely in the mist. Nearly everyone is unprepared to hear that bell. When we think about it, though, that wouldn't happen in the NFL or the NBA or the Olympics. So, why does it happen to us in life? What do successful athletes do that we do not?

NFL players spend the preseason and all year practicing strategies for the last two minutes, for the out-of-bounds plays that will stop the clock, for the onside kicks, and for those desperate fifty-yard field goals. NBA teams methodically practice strategies year-round for inbounding the ball under pressure with the seconds counting down to set up the last shot at the buzzer. When writing a final grade-determining term paper, you wouldn't wait until the last minute to start doing your research, developing an outline, and crafting your prose. So, why do you wait to do the research, outline your goals, and start pursuing them when your life and legacy are at stake?

If you are unprepared to hear the bell and stumble at the sound, you can still catch up if you have some clues what to expect. There is a great deal of pain that can suck the very happiness out of your days if you don't.

If there is anything good about cancer, it is that there is a bell and it is loud.

Alarm bells have been used for eons to call those within earshot to think and act. In medieval times, long before the telegraph, telephone or email, steeple bells were used to communicate and send specific messages across the countryside. When the ominous cadence of the Nine Tailors rang out, those huge, somber low pitched bells announced a death in the community. Today, it is the ICU alarm that sounds when electrical activity from a patient's heart arrests. However, when an aneurysm blows, a heart suddenly stops, or an unexpected catastrophe strikes, there is no warning bell. Game over! When dementia or Alzheimer's surreptitiously steals away life as we have known it, there has been no sounding bell and there is no chance for a bell lap. With cancer there is both a bell and a chance, so don't miss them—nor the small, but significant blessing they bring.

Your Biggest Hurdle

People seldom choose to talk about death. But the Dragon is already talking about death in your head and manipulating your thoughts with it—whether you recognize and admit it or not. The Dragon would just as soon you wouldn't talk about it so it can go about its vile business unimpeded. *You don't have to expect to die soon, but you do need to think about it.* Talking about death is a hurdle that everyone must clear in order to run a good bell lap. If not, their fear will get them running in the wrong direction. When death does creep into our thoughts, many wish for it to come quickly and painlessly—a blissful and anxiety free ending. The allure of such an exit is easy to see, but it is fraught with seldom considered downsides.

Few of us are really ready for death. Few have fully realized their purpose, fulfilled every commitment, transmitted every bit of accrued wisdom to the next generation, and celebrated it all until every tear has fallen and every cheering voice has grown hoarse. Although many think they are ready, few really are.

> **Curiously, it is those who are indeed ready to die who are actually the most ready to fully live.**

Death can be blissful and anxiety free, but not because of what goes on in your body. It has to do with what has already gone on in your head and heart—that is where you defeat the Dragon. Let's size up this hurdle and get over it, so an undistracted you can run an amazing lap while helping the doctors clobber the cancer.

Don't Waste Your Cancer

A friend was riding up the Rainier Express at the Crystal Mountain Ski Resort in the Cascade Mountains when a man skiing down the Sunnyside run right beneath the chairlift caught his eye. The skier was strong, agile, and obviously having a marvelous time. Suddenly, something went terribly wrong and he went careening helplessly down the hill like a ragdoll until a steep mogul arrested his descent. Some biologic event—a plug of platelets in a coronary artery, a quirk of electrical activity in his heart muscle, ventricular fibrillation, or a blown aneurysm in his brain suddenly ended his life—tragic for a sixty-six-year-old man who was obviously thoroughly engaged in the zest of living. I don't know the rest of his story, but I do know the passionate response of the guys sipping beer later and listening to it. "What a great way to go amid the exhilaration of a challenging adventure!"

It occurred to me, should my biology afford me an opportunity for such a rapid exit, how great it would be to have it come while skiing the steeps in deep powder on a cold sunny day—one minute in ecstasy and then in a heartbeat wake up in heaven.

Would I really be ready?
Would I have learned all that I needed or wanted to learn?
Would I have fulfilled all the responsibilities and opportunities of the life I've been given?
Would I really be in heaven?

With cancer there is a bell and there is a bell lap. There is time to plan and to get ready. If you run in the right direction, there will be enough time to complete it–and well. However, for those who choose not to run, there is never enough time. I know because I have watched some refuse to hear the bell. Others deny what it means and just run the wrong direction. Some give up and start dying the very day the bell rings, becoming like the walking dead who squander their remaining days in denial and despair instead of living each one fully until the last.

This is not a book about dying, it's about living. Some who read these words will die soon and some will not die for many years, but they both need to pay attention. Those who read these words, consider them, and take them to heart can live a fuller, more rewarding and exciting life. Maybe, just maybe, they can live a longer one as well.

Watch and Learn

Tim McGraw's lyrics, "live like you were dying," as trite as they may sound, are actually true. When they are followed, they produce extraordinary vitality. There is much to learn from watching those who know they are dying. The ones who collapse on the track do so either because they are totally unprepared or overwhelmed with fear or in total denial. Usually terror-ridden or distracted, they haven't given death a thought. The media emphasizes how awful, painful, ugly, and inglorious dying is and cultivates fear, disdain, and avoidance. Most religions have something to say about it, but they don't agree on how to prepare for it. There is not one of us who wouldn't like to know the rest of the story beyond death. The Bible has something to say, but it is seldom read or seriously considered. Even the pulpit devotes little effort to our society's biggest taboo subject.

Preparing Doesn't Hurt

We know from a study at Stanford University[1] that if you are far away from death—at least twenty years—you basically act as if you are immortal, as if you are going to live forever. That leaves most of us unprepared for death. At the sounding of the Bell when death raises its ugly head, it finds us bewildered.

Why is it we don't prepare for our bell lap?

What does preparation look like?

When should we start?

What resources do we need?

How do we make a plan and execute it?

Does it make a difference?

Does fixing our eyes beyond the finish line mean giving up fighting for life?

Is it the length of the lap, or how we run it or the lives we touch that is important?

How can we conceive a strategy when we don't know how long the bell lap will be?

My goal here is to help you answer these questions with the answers that best suit your temperament and circumstance, as well as how best to engage the medical community for the best biologic outcome. Those who formulate their own answers run better and longer during their final lap. They feel better about answering these questions once they reach the finish line.

What did you do with your last lap?
Did you really live it or were you just alive?

Get Prepared

What do you do when a storm-driven sailboat snaps its mast and runs aground or a climber gets high-altitude pulmonary edema and falls into a crevasse? What if your car crashes off a bridge into the water or you are lost in the mountains or in the desert without water and shelter? What if you are on a plane and the pilot has a heart attack? The Boy Scouts left an indelible mark on me with the motto, "Be Prepared." I have been preparing for every calamity my patients might face in the hospital or I might face in the wilderness–still working on how to ditch the plane if a pilot collapses–and I am diligently preparing how to live my life if I ever get cancer. Learning from others who have survived calamities at sea, in the mountains, and in front of bears has saved my bacon more than once.

I have come face to face with a charging grizzly bear, naked, defenseless, and scared, feeling just a little prepared. I have been overboard miles off shore alone with only my shorts–cold, scared, and again, just a little prepared. I have been by the side of friends facing death from cancer who were scared and totally unprepared. So, I have paid a lot of attention to the folks in peril who were prepared in order to learn and then teach from their stories. Sometimes, the face of cancer isn't a lot different from that of a growling bear. So, we will deal with cancer first and leave the bear for later.

To possess emotional and spiritual fortitude in a moment of crisis, takes forethought, training, and practice. Not surprising, if you train for the greatest crisis of them all, facing death (or a grizzly), you become more prepared for all the other crises of life as well. If death loses its sting, then how much sting can losing a job, a relationship or a leg have? Is it really possible to confront all these awful things with equanimity and not become crazy, out of touch, or numb? What does that look like and feel like? While they never feel good, they don't need to overwhelm or destroy us.

Getting prepared for the bell lap can change your perspective on a lot of things— indeed on life itself.

Leave the Plates on the Floor

Many of us have become Vaudevillian plate spinners with our lives, skilled at getting several plates in the air spinning at once, even making it look easy. We skillfully balance work, marriage, kids, more work, avocations, more kids, sports, aging parents, and community responsibilities. Enter illness and the plates come tumbling down. At first, we tremble and think it's our life that lays broken on the floor, but it is only our spinning plates. It is not the *Who* of what we are, only the *What* of who we were trying to be. Most of those who endure a serious illness, escape vaudeville and decide not to pick up all the plates when their health returns. One high school friend said how much cancer had changed his life for the better twenty years ago and lamented how he wished he had stuck with the changes. Temptations and the years had eroded what he had learned.

Some patients discover that their self-centered, constructed identities are only all-consuming charades, and their lists of perceived necessities are only media manufactured mirages. Often, they choose to leave most of it behind. Many experience sweet deliverance from those delusions through their encounter with illness. With their awakening, they are thankful that they heard the bell and many are even thankful for it.

The energy it takes to keep the plates spinning had taken a slickly veiled toll on their hearts, their families, and their lives.

Many had come to treasure their encounter with illness for the bittersweet release it had brought them from society's market-driven, self-centered seductions and necessities. Running the bell lap is not about getting more plates in the air, it's not about doing anything or being everything. It is simply about running the personal race set before us and passing on our own batons of wisdom and experience to those whom we will someday leave behind. Even though few are expecting departure soon, it compels preparation if one is to avoid either failure or anxiety.

Preparation starts with dropping some of the plates without feeling guilty or inadequate.

Procrastinating Is Normal, but Never Helpful

The cancer bell never rings at the right time or when it is convenient. Unlike a foot race where the bell rings after a predictable number of laps, we can seldom anticipate the bell announcing our last lap. Usually, we are caught off guard; we're not ready for it. If you think about it, we are seldom ready for life's major events. We choose the day for our weddings, but are we really ready? When it is time to choose a career and work for a living, are we ready? We discover we are pregnant and we just aren't ready. There is no perfect time, so don't put off getting prepared for each phase of the lap. You may already have been caught off guard by the diagnosis, but if you are reading this, you still have some of the lap ahead of you and you can start preparing for it.

All of us have lived our lives with deadlines. Ever since fifth grade when my first term paper became due, I have been faced with deadlines, met anxiety, and said *hello* to consequences. The classrooms of life have been no less brutal. Many of us have been so distracted by the exigencies and the delights, the gottas and wannas of life, that we have prepared little for our final exam, i.e. facing death. It may seem a stretch to make such a comparison, but the final draft is the one our children and our family will best remember. They will be reading it in their heads again and again after we are gone, indelible visual and auditory memories that can linger with privileged primacy. So it is with the bell lap. It can rewrite, redefine or accentuate an entire life. If a term paper is better written with preparation, so too is the bell lap. The bell is a reminder that it is time to plan and polish the final draft – and pray you will have the time and discipline to act it out.

Look It in the Face

This book is about living freely and to the fullest. However, to do that well one must ponder death. Even if your treatment regimen stands a high likelihood of curing you, do this anyway. You will never regret it and I promise you will be better off for having done so. It won't mean trying, hoping or believing any less in a cure. Just do it with me–now.

For eons, philosophers have been struggling to understand death and to overcome its gripping fear. Years after starting hospice and caring for countless patients facing death or skirting around its edges, I came across the printed words of an earlier mentor, Dr. Elizabeth Kubler Ross. They summarize just what those years have taught me: *"Death does not have to be a catastrophic, destructive thing; indeed it can be viewed as one of the most constructive, positive, and creative elements of culture and life"*[2]

When death is viewed as a thief in the night that steals away life, it can never be prepared for, let alone welcomed. It can only be feared. Some cultures make an overt effort to view it differently. Murray L. Trelease, a parish priest serving in the remote native villages in Alaska in the 1960s, had a chance to sit with natives who were dying. They practiced a hybrid of indigenous traditions and Christian beliefs brought in by missionaries. Before the introduction of modern medicine, their trajectory of illness toward death was more predictable. Today, by offering some degree of efficacy, treatment creates both hope and unpredictability. Without either of those back then, natives could more accurately foresee their death and developed rituals in which the dying would play an active, meaningful role for themselves and their community. Often the dying person would "spend days making plans, telling the story of his life, and praying for all the members of the family."[3]

There would often be some kind of formal gathering for celebration, prayers, farewells, and perhaps the Eucharist and hymns. The dying person would revel in this shower of affection. The activities were usually set in motion by the one dying, who sensed intuitively, "meaningful life was drawing to a close and was able to enter the final phase easily and naturally."[4] He/she didn't need a doctor to affirm terminality. Without the mysterious interventions of unpredictable medicines, natives were able to trust their intuitions. Frequently, death ensued very slowly thereafter, almost as if they willed it to be so.

**It seems there is much we can learn from those
so-called primitive people!**

Will to Live—A Power, a Delusion, or an Excuse?

My experiences with the seriously ill have convinced me that the will to live or its surrender can sometimes affect the number of our days and breaths. This is less profound in the era of modern medicine because medical interventions can play such a dramatically determinant role. However, the effect of the will is real and deserves attention and respect. Murray Trelease puts it well: "It is not that human will changes reality, but that it is a part of the reality of life and needs to be reckoned with." The intuition of the terminally ill needs to be cultivated, recognized, honored, and empowered. Well-intended modern medicine is quick to disregard the intuition and disenfranchise the will of the individual. Doctors will readily grab control if patients and families relinquish it. Recognize that modern medicine often seeks to optimize treatment with only survival in mind. It can blindly disregard the meaning and purpose of the life of the patient who must endure the long-term side effects of being "optimized."

Beware: Completing the bell lap well, with celebration, a good baton pass, personal healing, and many blessings is not the commission of modern medicine.

There comes a time when trusting your intuition is more important than trusting your physician's advice, no matter how expert and well-intentioned it may be. There is a time to decline a doctor's good intentions. Figuring out your priorities and how to shuffle them is your job. Doctors often do not offer much help in this arena.

Before the advances of current medicine, the outcome of an illness or injury was fairly predictable and little could be done to alter it. Now, that has changed and with that change has come a new tension in the gap between the possible and the inevitable, between fighting for survival and the acceptance of death.

The achievements of medical science have given us a greater sense of control over life-threatening illness and injury, which is both valid and delusional. It is valid in the scientific, biologic sense, but delusional in the existential sense. Medicine is not perfect, the possibility of dying too soon and the certainty of dying eventually are unchanged. The gap between the possible and the certain has widened, and in that gap, the Dragon flourishes.

The need to deal with the certainty of death has not been diminished one iota by science, only postponed—often until it is too late. The cost of that postponement is a haunting anxiety which may be blatantly destructive, like the subtle creeping dry rot in the hull of a ship. Some people fall apart immediately as if they hit a land mine, while others just fade away allowing the dry rot to eat away at what remains of their lives.

Addressing the death issue can be accomplished well and completely without surrendering hope or a single effort for a cure. It is accomplished more easily if done before it is staring you in the face.

Don't let the intoxicating hopes of modern medicine dissuade you from doing the necessary work in confronting the certainty of death. Yes, you can put off thinking about it, but at a cost which allows the Dragon room to roam. Instead, let me help you size up everything that you are up against, face it, deal with it, and overcome it. This will catapult you into what I hope will be a long and wonderful backstretch.

Windrunners To-Do List

- Hear the Bell
- Run in the Right Direction
- Start Preparing for the Whole Lap
- Leave Some Plates on the Floor

The First Stretch

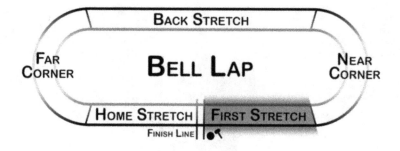

Chapter 2

Winning Means Knowing What You Are Up Against

"If you die that does not mean you lose to cancer. You beat cancer by how you live, why you live, and in the manner in which you live. So live. Live. Fight like hell and when you get too tired to fight, then lay down and rest and let someone else fight for you."[6]

Don't allow the disease to dictate how you live. It is in the strength and beauty of the human spirit to never give up. Don't let the disease dictate what you are living for; it's about more than just staying alive. Running the bell lap involves many things. Some are pragmatic, some frivolous, some mundane, and some intriguing. Others are physical, some spiritual, and a few are just for you while some are just for others. They are all laced with uncertainty: uncertain energy, uncertain resources, and uncertain time available. It is all infused with urgency and often with confusion, especially as to where to begin.

The bell lap of your race is like any high-stakes race in an oval track stadium. It may not be your last lap, but because it might be, you had better treat it as if it is. You are the only one on the track, while everyone else is in the stands. When the bell rings, your first thought will usually jump ahead to winning the race or just plain surviving. Those thoughts are a distraction. Your life is not immediately threatened even though it may feel that way. You should really be thinking about what is right in front of you and what it is going to take to get you into the first corner in the inside lane for the shortest, most direct path to remission in the backstretch. If you blow the race in the first stretch by focusing on the finish line, it is hard to play catch-up.

The first stretch is key, and to run it well you need to have some sense of what you are up against in the whole race:

- The condition of the track (the whole medical menagerie).
- The characteristics of your opponents (the cancer and the Dragon).
- An assessment of your own fitness (physical, social, emotional, and spiritual).

What Does this Race Look Like?

A running track is typically divided into five sections that are useful in planning race strategy. In life's run with cancer, we can use these sections to help us understand better what this race is going to look like.

1) The First Stretch: The confusing period of testing, prognosticating, and rearranging your life.

2) The Near Corner: The hard times of initiating treatment and confronting the adversaries to your heart.

3) The Backstretch: The perplexing times of maintenance treatment and wondering what to do with remission and the rest of your life.

4) The Far Corner: The worrisome times dealing with relapse treatment decisions while completing the baton pass.

5) The Homestretch: The unavoidable times of anticipating death.

Looking over the whole course, including the far corner and homestretch which are hopefully far off, will help you run the earlier sections better. Most likely the ringing bell didn't give you a chance to do that, so do it now and adjust your run down the first stretch accordingly. When you do, you'll discover you are in a whole new environment of medicine. You are confronted with both a disease (what cancer can do to your body) and an illness (what cancer and its treatment can do to your life), and you are reeling from the possible amputation of the future you thought you had.

What Kind of Track Shoes Do You Need?

Those who ignore their souls (shoes) never run well. They falter and stumble and eventually drop out of the running. Winners choose a matched pair carefully. For this particular race, the right shoe is called "hope," and the left is called "acceptance." Those who have run this race successfully will tell you that you can't really run well with only one; both are equally important. They must be used sequentially and that takes both coaching and practice. Neither is as easy as it sounds and both are more important than one would imagine. There are nuances of each that apply to every segment of the lap which, when understood and addressed, will make your run easier, faster, and longer.

**You are confronted with a *disease*—
what cancer can do to your body.
You are also confronted with an *illness*—
what cancer and treatment can do to your life.**

There might be a surprise competitor in this race and it might be you—the other you, the one who doesn't figure out what winning really looks like. It's about more than just surviving. Most don't figure it out until half way down the backstretch and that is okay. Some don't even try. They arrogantly respond with an earthy scatological, "I want my old life back and right now!" However, that is not one of the options. Your body is going to change and so is your life whether you want it to or not. The only question is how and in what direction, and a lot of that is up to you.

Humor me on this and try to remain open to discovering what I'm talking about. Let me teach you how to run this race you never wanted to enter. Let me review with you what many winners have done—when, why, and how. Then you can pick up whatever tips fit your circumstances and come up with your own plan.

Winners don't collapse on the track at the sound of the bell, nor do they turn tail and run in the wrong direction. They take off for the near corner, pushing aside for the moment all thoughts of, "Can I really do this?" This can be done! You can chose the best treatment and take it. You can turn down worthless stuff that is offered despite the good intentions of the offeree. I am going to help you.

All winners do three things:

1) Every morning they put on both shoes and focus on their particular illness and what it can do to their particular life.

2) They get to know the track; that strange new environment into which their disease has plummeted them.

3) They start planning and dreaming about where they want their life to go in spite of their illness.

They also do a fourth thing—they forgive their bodies, their God, themselves, and their cancer. Getting sidetracked blaming or establishing fault is a self-defeating strategy. Getting stuck in unforgiveness can be an obsession on the road to victimhood and victims never win. Seeking justice and pity gets you nowhere. There will be things you will never understand. Until you accept that and forgive it all, you cannot get on with winning. We want to identify everything you can control so you can get equipped to control them. Then we want to also identify those things you can't control so you can find a way over, around or through them.

Ultimately, the strategy for the bell lap comes down to identifying the factors you can control or at least influence, and going after them while letting go of the rest.

Winning Means Knowing Your Environment

The language and terminology of medicine is foreign to most of us. It's strange and often contains disgusting topics, new

46

interpersonal dynamics, machines, needles, tubes, and smells that are different from anything we have ever had to face prior to beginning this race. We must take the time to learn about this new environment we are being thrust into if we want to win this race.

If you don't understand the environment, each portion of it is a potential source of uncertainty and fear that the Dragon can exploit against you. Every unknown that you can eliminate now is one less that you will have to deal with later, and one less burden on your back as you come running into the backstretch. You must start off by learning as much about your new environment as possible by pummeling the nurses and staff with every question you can think of. They are usually savvy and can expand on what the doctor has said or what you forgot to ask.

Survivors in the wild try to understand their environment before a crisis arrives. This applies as much for patients in the foreign terrain of a cancer hospital as it is for climbers in the mountains or sailors on the ocean. Loving risky adventures, I read *Deep Survival,* by Lawrence Gonzales, to prepare for the next calamity I might encounter. I wanted to glean whatever tips I could from true survivors about how to improve my odds out in the wilderness. If ever I find myself at the bottom of a crevasse with a broken leg, adrift in the open ocean in a dingy or being chased by bear, I want to know that someone else has survived the same predicament and just how they did it. That is what you want to know from cancer survivors and exactly what I want to tell you.

Gonzales recounts amazing stories of disaster survival. He studied those who survived and those who did not, and discovered what behaviors distinguished the two. He points out how frequently climbing or hunting parties are made up of mostly followers and just one leader. Followers follow. They allow themselves to be disconnected from their environment, not taking in the visual and auditory cues that identify where they are, never alert to what distinguishes each turn in the path. Followers are simply "going along for the ride" like passengers in a car or *passive patients in a cancer clinic*. The followers are the folks who, when on their own, are really lost, out of touch, couldn't cope, and didn't survive.

**Having cancer is a lonely business.
You have got to be paying attention because
no one else is walking in your shoes.**

In survival school, everyone learns to walk their own walk and not blindly go along with the crowd. They are taught to watch the sky for weather changes, monitor the wind and temperature, and frequently turn around to look at the back trail. The way home looks completely different facing in the opposite direction, especially in the fog, at night or under stress. The way out will be unrecognizable if not studied going in. It is important to create a mental map of your journey with distinct waypoints that you will be able to identify when trying to find your way home.

In order for you to survive the cancer and your illness, I want to teach you how to interact with your new environment. I want to tune you into the changes in your body, soul, and spirit, and to anticipate what to expect from friends and family. I want to teach you about the doctors—who they are, what motivates them, and what limits them. I want to help you make a mental map of expectations and experiences as you are likely to travel similar paths/treatments more than once, quite possibly amidst confusion and stress.

If you learn this, you will feel more in control, more able to lead a fuller life, and do better with your treatment. At the beginning, you will be told about a bewildering list of possible side effects, but you may not be told when to expect them or the real likelihood of their occurrence. Some people are so overwhelmed that they just check out. Others enter a perpetual state of anxiety, fearing that at any moment any or all of the side effects will occur. The Dragon is quick to exploit and compel such people to hibernate at home to avoid even the risk of unpleasant side effects in public. All of a sudden, life gets very small; but there is a better way.

Winners To-Do List

- Every morning put on both shoes: "hope" and "acceptance."
- Get to know the track: the cancer clinic and all the staff.
- Start planning and dreaming about where you want your life to go in spite of your illness.
- Identify everything you can control.

Chapter 3

Winning Means Knowing Your Environment

Doctors have their own special style and language for talking to you. You need to have your own for talking to them, as well.

You cannot leave the starting blocks without learning the type, grade, and stage of your particular cancer. At the outset, everyone may have a notion of what cancer and cancer treatment is, but it is highly unlikely that your concept aligns with your specific type and stage of cancer.

Cancer is a behavioral disease of cells the way crime is a behavioral disorder of humans. Cells which have become cancerous have two aberrant, neigh criminal, behaviors: uncontrolled multiplication and a proclivity to spread to other parts of the body.

Normal cells respect their neighbors and do not multiply when there is no room or need for repair, whereas cancer cells keep multiplying taking up precious space and taking over the local blood and oxygen supply until neighboring normal cells die or are crowded out. At any point, cancer cells may break away to travel in the blood stream or lymph channels (tiny channels like veins that carry lymph fluid instead of blood) to other parts of the body where they settle in like squatters and start multiplying and taking over again. Polite normal breast cells stay in the breast, whereas malignant/cancerous ones can travel/metastasize to many other places (most commonly lymph nodes, bones, and liver, but also skin and lung, but rarely the brain) and start making trouble there.

There are as many *types of cancer as there are cell types in the body*. The type of cancer is determined by where the cancer started, not by which organ it has spread to. Location does not change the type. For example, World War II started in Germany and later spread to France, Russia, and North Africa. The enemy was always the Nazis. Like the enemy in World War II, each type of cancer occurs in a whole spectrum of *grades* and *stages*. *Grade* is how aggressive the cancer is (Nazi Storm Troopers versus drafted German citizens). *Stage* characterizes the extent of spread of the cancer through the body.

Nazism was a malignant behavior of humans. When Nazism was just growing in Germany, it was like a Stage I cancer. When it spread to Poland, it became like a Stage II cancer, which has spread from its primary site to the adjacent lymph nodes. When it spread by air or water to North Africa and Norway, it became like the highest stage, a Stage IV cancer, which spread through the blood stream to the liver, lungs, brain or bone.

Each type of cancer has a different form of treatment, modified according to its grade, stage, and genetics, or cell surface characteristics.

Ask Your Doctor about Prognosis Repeatedly

Prognosis tells you what to expect in terms of length of life only *as of that moment.* It will change as time passes and new information comes in, as your cancer responds to treatment or not and how well and how fast. So you must ask repeatedly. Initially, doctors should give you an estimate how long you will live if you take no treatment to give you a baseline against which you can consider treatment.

Researchers study hundreds or thousands of patients with your specific type, grade, and stage of cancer and average their findings to provide estimates how long the average patient will live with or without various treatments. Your doctor will use those averages to generate your prognosis. You are not necessarily average, so your doctor can often adjust the prognosis somewhat based upon your unique circumstances. Even after that has been done, you need to know that there are patients who will, for as yet unknown reasons, do dramatically better or worse than the averages. There may also be new treatments discovered during your lifetime which may change your prognosis altogether. These are rare, so you cannot build your plans for the bell lap on those, but they are good to put in your hope chest.

So ask these questions:

1. What is the average survival of someone with *my* stage of *my* cancer with no treatment at all or with the same treatments available to me?

2. What is the long term/short term survival range? Is there anything special about my circumstances that suggest I may be more toward one end of the survival range or another?

3. If my cancer is thought to be incurable, i.e., Stage IV, and my present cancer symptoms are not interfering with living my life, what difference would it make if the starting of treatment were delayed until symptoms appear or worsen? What would the absolute difference in the length my survival be as measured in months or years?

4. If the difference isn't much, could I delay treatment which would allow me to go on with my life unaltered by treatment side effects? Would such a delay likely result in otherwise avoidable symptoms that could be more difficult to control later?

Doctors speak most about RR (response rates), DFS (disease-free survival rates), and OS (overall survival rates).These are important metrics, but don't answer the above nitty gritty questions which you need answered in order to plan your life and bell lap. The RR is the rate that a given treatment will result in tumor response (shrinkage) as either a PR (partial response, which is 50 percent tumor shrinkage), or a CR (complete response which is complete disappearance of all cancer on physical exam, scans, and blood markers). RR equals PRs plus CRs. Unfortunately, CR does not equal the cure rate! Unfortunately, we have no test to measure the presence or absence of every last tiny, tiny cancer cell which may be hidden beyond the sensitivity of our tests and could regrow later.

The smallest tumor mass we can detect contains about 500 million cancer cells. This means there can be innumerable masses smaller than that which can go undetected with even our best scans even in someone who has achieved a CR. Doctors start talking about cure rates only in those individuals who achieve a CR and remain in CR for a number of years, sometimes after two years in the case of fast-growing cancers, or after five to ten years for slower growing ones.

When they can't talk about cure, they can talk about MDR or median duration of remission. This is roughly the average time that any remission will last before new or growing cancer can be detected requiring a change of treatment. During this time, one may be off treatment altogether or on maintenance medication. One must recognize that the MDR is only an average. Any individual's remission may be shorter or longer. At least knowing the average gives one some information for planning life.

Get Your Prognosis in Detail

Your next set of questions is designed to give you a more detailed prognosis so you can begin to plan out your bell lap.

Ask your doctor what impact he expects your disease will have on:

- the length and quality of your life
- your ability to work
- your ability to think clearly
- your ability to eat, sleep, and play

Pin him down. Ask specifically for both the worst and the best scenarios. You will probably be given a range for each one. Note: Prognosis and response rates to treatment are different.

Beware of the physician who softens the truth about your prognosis, either in an attempt to help you cope or to make his day easier. It does you no favor if it deprives you of the real, albeit discouraging, news that can motivate you to make the most of your dwindling resource of time. Insist on knowing the worst possible outcome, as that is what you need to be prepared for. Fantasies are short lived and always disappointing. Accept the worst just for now, (we'll talk about bettering the best later) and start making a plan for how to deal with it meaningfully.

Beware of your physician's prognosis *and* beware of what you think the physician is saying about your prognosis. As patients, we tend to have selective hearing, choosing what we want to hear, and physicians tend to be selective in speaking, carefully choosing specific words to protect your feelings. Both doctors and patients tend to excel at giving and receiving good news, but are lousy at giving and receiving grave news. Often times, the prognosis is a combination of both some good and some bad. It is likely the good will be exaggerated and the bad will be glossed over in both the delivery and the reception. Beware.

It is imperative to listen carefully and ask questions incisively. For the emotionally fragile individual, the possibility of any unfavorable side effect can be so frightening that they will be scared away from a therapy with some significant chance of benefit. Therefore, doctors choose their words carefully and don't exaggerate. Yet, a careful explanation of the downside risks is necessary in order for a patient to be prepared should such risks occur. The doctor/patient conversation is a dance. Don't scare them too much, but tell them just enough to prepare them and avoid the accusation "you never told me about xyz."

We are all fragile, and only you, not the doctor, know how much. Physicians are good at managing disease, but you are best at managing your life. Do not assume these are the same, because they aren't. You will need to coax the untold truth about your prognosis and risks out of your doctor. He will be afraid of diminishing the hope that sustains you, thus, may inadvertently leave you with a false hope, hence unprepared. The only way to avoid allowing false hopes to influence your decisions is to not need them. Only unshakable truths that are independent of treatment outcome can give you real freedom (see *Windrunners and The Dragon Vanquished*). If you have those, your doctor can shoot straight with you and you will hear what he is really saying. Then you can avoid the consequences of misguided hope decisions.

What Is the Chance This Will Work?

This is a question you must ask should you relapse and want to consider more treatment. It is a time you must remember the critical differences between RR, PR, CR, OS, MDR, and Cure. You must listen carefully for which one the doctor is talking about. Beware when treatment is described as having some percentage chance of working *without "working" being defined.* It often only means OR=objective response. That is any measurable response or tumor shrinkage less than 50 percent, which may or may not be clinically meaningful to you in terms of quality or length of life (measurable but not beneficial). This distinction is extraordinarily important! The quality and even the quantity of your remaining life are at stake and can both be diminished.

Notice that a treatment which works only 10 percent of the time and produces only minor shrinkage isn't worth much and never cures or prolongs life. Sadly, here is where a common and unintended miscommunication often happens between physician and patient. The doctor says the treatment has some chance of "working," meaning "working at least a little," and the patient interprets "working" as working a lot, maybe for a long time, maybe even a cure. They see a glimmer of hope that they will return to their normal life, but that is not what the physician has said and indeed it never happens in such a situation.

It is essential to know that disease response, OR (Objective Response) and PR (Partial Response) do not necessarily increase the chance of prolonging life, let alone offer a cure. Some treatments may be worth attempting if they will decrease symptoms of the cancer. However, if the toxicity of the medicine is worse than the symptoms of the cancer, then the medicine may not be worth taking, especially if there is not a chance of cure or significant prolongation of quality life. So, ask and be clear. No doctor will be upset with your questions. Most likely they will be relieved to have the opportunity to be explicit.

Therefore, be certain you fully understand what the doctor is saying about expectations and toxicities before signing up for more treatment. This is usually not a critical issue when someone is contemplating their first line treatment or maybe even second line. But it is an absolutely critical issue when considering salvage third or fourth line treatment. If the doc says a treatment might work or you may respond, he may just be glossing over or avoiding talking about a dire reality by basically providing a placebo and a false hope. Remember, you are entitled to have every question answered in a way you understand. You may need to re-ask the question several times to get the answer you need; don't be bashful.

Family and friends need to know that when curative treatment stops, it doesn't mean that life will bounce back to exactly what it was pre-cancer. You will be different, physically, socially, and perhaps spiritually—in some ways better, some worse, but never the same.

Learn What to Expect

Treatment is often intermittent in cycles every three to six weeks for months on end. With radiation, it could be a continuous course lasting three to six weeks. You need not drop out of life completely to take treatment, but you will want to make some rational allowances for possible side effects. One of the most predictable is the loss of energy, but it is neither continuous nor uniform in severity.

Ask your doctor to draw you a timeline, or preferably a graph, with the days and weeks of the whole treatment course outlined on a horizontal "x-axis" and the severity of possible side effects on the vertical "y-axis." At one glance, it should show you when your blood counts will fall and rise, how your energy and sense of well-being will fluctuate, when mouth sores, diarrhea, fever, rash, numbness or tingling, etc. might occur (not to suggest they will because that depends on the drug, the dose, and your own unique biology), and when they would be expected to resolve. Then you can look at the timeline and see that there are blocks of time when side effects are likely to be minimal. That is when you can plan special events, get your workouts, do tasks, go to work, etc. You will also see other times when you shouldn't expect much of yourself, need to give yourself grace, should limit commitments, and recruit assistance in advance.

Unpredictability vs. Sense of Control

Living in unpredictability can be a nightmare and is often depressing. Knowing what to expect and having it in a visual/graphic form that you can refer back to after you've forgotten everything a doctor said will limit unpredictability, improve your sense of control, and lessen the likelihood of depression. If depression does set in, it can really sap your energy even further, as well as defeat any creativity and dissipate every passion. However, it doesn't have to be that way.

I advise patients that they are going to lose 20 percent of their energy overall with chemotherapy, some days more, some less. Most of us use 80 to 90 percent of our energy for the work and chores of life and use the leftover 10 to 20 percent for fun and meaningful stuff. There is a danger that, as energy declines, people will only have enough left for work and chores. Burnout beckons, relationships suffer, depression smolders, and the Dragon revels in its playground.

At the outset, I counsel patients to cut down their workload, both on the job and at home, by 20 percent to preserve enough time and energy for the essential things like relating to the kids, loving a spouse, meeting with friends, and pursuing avocations. Think of energy as currency: spend it now or save it for later—when it's gone, it is gone!

Offload responsibilities at home by recruiting the kids, spouse, friends, and family to pick up the slack in ways such as making meals, doing chores, paying the bills, etc. Celebrate high energy times by dining out. Grab an occasional takeout when energy levels are too low to cook. Be intentional about times for dating, playing, church, and family. Deny the Dragon a foothold by planning proactively and giving yourself the grace to delegate and ask for help. If you're doing better than expected, invest in yourself by exercising, reading, or spending time with friends, mentors, and counselors.

The stronger you are emotionally and spiritually, the stronger you can be physically to tolerate treatment. Improved tolerance translates to improved treatment and improved survival. When you make life better, it makes your life more worth fighting to save.

Winners To-Do List

- Know Exactly What You Are Up Against
- Ask Your Doctor about Prognosis
- Repeatedly Get Your Prognosis in Detail
- Learn What to Expect and Write it Down

Chapter 4

Winning Means Playing Your Part

Keep Your Own Records

The mountaineer looks back over his shoulder so he can find his way home at twilight. You need to look back and chart your experience by keeping records of your energy levels, the time course, and severity of every side effect through each treatment cycle. It will help your physician improve your treatment.

Many chemotherapy treatments consist of a combination of drugs, each of which has a different side effect profile. Depending upon which side effects you experience, he can decrease the amount of the offending drug and increase the amount of another inoffensive drug to maintain efficacy while decreasing toxicity at the same time. You win and cancer loses, but only if you are an astute observer, careful record keeper, and effective communicator of your symptoms.

These habits will also help you predict what to expect how to live during future treatment cycles, and will give you back some control over your life.

Better yet, recruit a partner on your team to accompany you and to do record keeping with you. Doing so unloads a responsibility enabling you to focus all your attention on understanding and digesting what is being said. It also creates a meaningful way for another to be involved in your life. It's not just a luxury, it is important; a friendly advocate at your side during appointments can also add volume to your voice when speaking to the doctors, spouse, and kids.

The illness experience can steal away your voice. The medical culture that applauds compliance, the time that is always too short, the turf that is foreign, and the invariable fatigue all conspire to silence patients. Figuring that the doctor knows best, patients strive for quiescent obedience. However, physicians cannot guess information that you haven't shared. With a friend at your side for courage, their memory for facts, their voice for volume, and your own good notes, effective advocacy for your health can prevail. By being a better patient, you can help your doctor be a better doctor and everyone gets a better outcome. When a physician and patient work together, remissions are longer and cures are more frequent.

As an overwhelmed patient, it is hard to be attuned to the gestures, the tone of voice, and the subtleties of language of the physician that are meant to span the gulf between what they say and what they really mean. Physicians are human and it can be hard for them to say what needs to be said. A partner at your side can observe and translate for you.

Confront the Illness

Illness and disease are not the same. Illness is what happens to your life when disease attacks your body. Do not confuse them. You have a role in dealing with both, but it is only the illness for which you have responsibility and over which you must take complete control. Recruit doctors to battle the disease and hand off most of that responsibility to them. Then find the wisdom to deal proactively with *your* illness as it impacts *your* life. Unmanaged, it can persist for years after the disease is in remission or cured.

Many mistakenly assume the illness will go away when the disease does; it doesn't.

The disease is an enemy that can be seen, felt, measured, and to a significant degree predicted, which gives the doctors a target for their attack. The illness is none of those things, yet it can be every bit as destructive. It can only be measured by the absence of joy, peace, and purpose in your life and relationships. It cannot be eliminated, but it can be understood, outsmarted, and overcome. With determination, anyone can do it, and with style.

Doctors fight disease with medicines, whereas you must take on illness with ideas. Doctors send you to the pharmacy for medicine, but I am sending you to mentors to learn how they think. Don't confuse your role with the physician's. Some patients get sidetracked focusing on treating their disease themselves with diets, potions, ablutions, abstentions, and all kinds of stuff, wasting time and energy that could be focused on their illness, which is threatening to overwhelm their lives and take them out. There is not much point in being physically alive if the life you are trying to lead is dead and gone. Direct your attention at the illness—find it, reveal it, expose it, and overcome it.

Save your life. Let the doctors save your body.

What Worked for Other Survivors?

In *Deep Survival*, Lawrence Gonzales describes a couple of different castaways. Stephen Callahan, a solo Atlantic sailor, was awakened by a loud crashing sound from what must have been a whale striking the hull of his sloop. What followed was gushing, cold saltwater, and lots of it. In another event, Debbie Kirby was a crew member on a 58 foot ketch which also sank, but in a hurricane. Separated in time and miles apart, each found themselves in a life raft equipped with little except the will to live and an exorbitant amount of sun, wind, water, and time. Gonzales analyzed and catalogued what enabled Callahan and Kirby to survive alone for months in the open ocean and it applies to surviving months in cancer treatment.

He found that Callahan "was orderly. He set about small tasks. He took responsibility to get them done and focused tightly and then he rested."[6] He never lost his sense of humor. In his diary he recorded, "I continue to make light of whatever I can in order to relieve the tension."[7] Patients I have known attest that humor is better than any drug—it has no side effects save laughter. Gonzales concluded, "Gratitude, humility, wonder, imagination, and cold logical determination were the survivor's tools. [8] But it was the dreams that were the motivation and the refuge—indeed, their only refuge from stark reality. Dreams are important and dreams about one's plans and purpose are huge.

Most of us have constructed busy lives for ourselves. When illness intervenes, our ability to pursue those lives becomes impaired, and many dreams die. The very things that have given our lives the most meaning may no longer be possible. We can feel disenfranchised from life, devalued, and lose our identity and purpose for living. We are left with only a bald-faced, self-centered quest for survival. Monotony can settle in, while adventure and purpose seep away. If you don't get intentional about finding your purpose and/or adventure, the monotony can become a wicked culture medium for incubating depressing thoughts and suicide. Purpose and possibility can and must be restored. Rick Warren observes, "Without purpose life has no meaning. The greatest tragedy is not death, but life without purpose." Furthermore, "when life has meaning you can bear most anything; without it, nothing is bearable."[9]

Focusing and Balancing Your Efforts

Even while dealing with the hard stuff after the bell rings, find some time for focused, purposeful dreaming. It is fun, important, and it sets up running the backstretch. Do not make it about forever, but only about today, this week, and next month. We will address forever later, but that cannot be the focus of the first stretch. You can't focus on hitting the ball out of the park until you focus on hitting the ball.

To begin with, dreams need to be focused around the worst prognosis your doctors have given you so you can be certain they are achievable. You don't have to like the doctor's prognosis, and you don't have to give up on hope, stamina, grit or prayer, nor the determination to prove them wrong. You do not have to accept that imminent death is certain or eventual death is probable, but you do need to accept that what they say and even death are possible.

You have got to give that idea more than just lip service. You need to let it settle into your heart so that it can change the way you think and act. If you let it sink in, it will hurt, but it doesn't have to be crippling. You are already entertaining the possibility of death in some measure every day when you put on your seatbelt. Buckling up doesn't mean you plan to be in a car accident, but it does mean that you are accepting the fact that a car accident is possible and that you are going to act accordingly. Focusing your dreams within the confines of your doctor's worst prognosis does not mean you are giving up, wimping out or planning to die, but that you are taking the prognosis seriously every day until it doesn't happen.

If you don't accept your doctor's worst prognosis as at least possible for the purposes of planning and dreaming, you invite the Dragon to draw near enough to get his claws of denial and fear into your back. I've never seen anyone run well, and I mean no one, who has those two on their back, denial and fear, clawing at their neck and whispering that foul breath in their ear. You can't focus all your energy on survival if you are expending it dealing with the Dragon or take flight to fantasy land to avoid it.

A sense of tragedy is unavoidable when it looks like life might end unfinished, but endings can be rewritten by those who are willing to dream and try. It takes courage, and that is not something you are born with; it is something you develop. It takes both hope and acceptance to do so, but it creates more of each in return.

Hope Is Critical—Right Foot

Many stumble in the first stretch. It is only hope that can pick them up off the track and get them going again. It is hope that provides the fuel to power them through the near corner. Somewhere beyond pain and despair there is hope. Find the courage to embrace it. For now, it is better to just grab onto some hope and know that it is real, than to spend much time searching for every last bit you can find. You need your eyes for something else. If you focus too much on fortifying all your hopes right now, you can become blind to the presence of the adversaries on the track which, if unseen, can knock you out of the running. This is a big deal. Pay attention! Grab onto some hope, and then turn your attention fully to the tasks of running the first stretch and the near corner. When you get to the backstretch, we will get to know every flavor of hope intimately and let them be the inspiration that enables you to run and finish well, whether in the near or distant future.

Accepting – Left Foot

Many patients tell me that achieving what they hope for and accepting what they need to accept is very hard to do on their own. Some try, some don't. Some ask God for help, some don't. Some are surprised to experience peace, some never do. It always takes time and it always hurts. I am told that starting to work on it early lessens the pain in the long run.

There are actually blessings to be found in almost every illness. Without trivializing illness or the changes it imposes on your life, I encourage you to seek out the possible upsides. Whining about your misfortune, no matter how justified, will not bring you happiness, but recognizing the positives will. One is the effect illness has on time. It creates it and with new time comes opportunity. Impudently, illness interrupts routines, making some planned events impossible. Giving those up can be hard, but when you do, it creates spaces in an otherwise packed agenda. That new unscheduled time may be the in-between times while waiting for appointments or the flaked-out times in bed when you are alert, but simply too tired or disabled to work or play. These are times you can either seethe with frustration or you can cut yourself some slack, sit back, read, and think things over or pray.

Wow! That contemplative time you never seemed able to find is now yours. You may not want it, but you've got it, so use it and put it to your benefit.

Another blessing is a new legitimate opportunity to unload some of your self-imposed or otherwise assigned, responsibilities. Grab it. Get rid of some stuff. The world will not stop. Life will go on. Your family will survive. You're not nearly as critical as you think you are at work or at home. You are important, worthy, and lovable, but probably not critical. On the other hand, figuring out the rest of your life's priorities and purpose is a critical responsibility. Planning your bell lap is crucial. Illness creates the moments, the opportunities, and the motivation to do just that. Don't miss them. Go for it.

Family Planning

There are growing numbers of patients surviving cancer. For young patients, part of planning for life after cancer may include family planning. This needs to be undertaken in the first stretch as soon as possible. Not all treatments impair fertility long-term and none have been shown to produce birth defects in children conceived three months after a completed treatment. While on treatment practicing sex is okay, but conceiving babies is not. Act accordingly. For those treatment regimens that do cause long-term sterility, pre-treatment sperm storage or storage of eggs or embryos can be undertaken before treatment begins. The storage procedure takes time, so it must be initiated immediately. Most cancers grow so slowly that treatment can be delayed somewhat for storage to take place. For those couples who are sexually active, contraception is in order and techniques may need to change. Lubrication becomes an issue, especially for the seniors on the circuit. Get professional advice rather than leave the game. Cancer doctors are notoriously bashful in this arena, perhaps even inept, but gynecologists and pharmacists are not. Many of my patients got the most help from the staff at the local love pantry store, as well as some blushing entertainment and education.

Slow Down and Take Your Time

When the chance of survival is uncertain and the prospect of a dramatic change in the course of life is just too scary to consider, some simply refuse to read the writing on the wall. Instead, they hunker down and plow ahead, taking on more and more, moving ever faster and faster, burning themselves up and others out. At such speed, wisdom cannot be found and her whispers are rarely heard, but the Dragon will not remain silent, in fact he will cheer you on.

Cancer itself is not evil; bodies do break down, but the Dragon will use cancer as a tool to do evil things in your life, the most destructive of which is to poison your attitudes. Sure, cancer can change life as you know it by spoiling dreams and hopes. However, when the Dragon can convince you that your present life, dreams, and hopes are the only ones worth considering, and when he sets you avariciously clinging to them, you become more likely to lose them or live in perpetual fear of losing them. There are other dreams that are magnificent and other hopes that are unshakeable beyond the reach of the Dragon. Go find them.

The Dragon will try to dishearten and distract you. He will try to keep your focus on what you are losing rather than on what you might gain. He may even try to convince you it isn't worth the effort to search for those other dreams and hopes. But you are in control; don't drink that poison.

Tomorrow's dreams are seldom constructed on the run. So slow down, figure out what dreams you should let go of or at least put on hold, then dream some new ones that you can hang on to. Dreams are essential motivators. I remember too well that it was only by helping my exhausted seven-year-old son fantasize about a cheeseburger and a hot fudge sundae that enabled him to walk out of the woods from the fishing trip planned by his overzealous father, and it was those same dreams that help me carry him when his legs gave out.

Dream boldly (right foot), but hold your dreams with a loose grip (left foot).

In nearly every recorded saga of extraordinary survival, the protagonist describes the importance of dreaming, even fantasizing about hopeful future events. Whether it was those stranded in a lifeboat out on ocean, a POW in a solitary cell, or others lost on a high Peruvian glacier after a plane crash, those who survived were all dreamers. It enabled them to do whatever they had to in order to survive. Dreams need not be big; indeed, many smaller ones are often better.

You may be lost in an otherworldly spell of a serious illness, but just because illness has blown old dreams into smithereens, don't let it be a black hole that sucks in every new dream. Don't let it paralyze you. Conjure up new ones within the limitations of your prognosis. Make them audacious, plan them out, and start running after them. Let them compel you forward and give you purpose. Set goals that are obtainable. Write them down. Make a list. It will surprise you when you begin to accomplish one goal at a time.

Don't permit cancer to dictate how you live. Don't let it disable you by getting you focused on what you can't do. Instead, focus on what you can do now, and do it before your next nap. Then applaud yourself when you've done it, plan again, and nap again.

If there is something important that seems out of reach, recruit someone to help. The list should include inactive things as well as active things, things you can do on your own and those for which you will need help, things that cost nothing and maybe things that cost a lot. Recruit a helpmate, spouse, sibling, child or a friend to brainstorm dreaming with you.

Ideally, recruit one or two people to run the bell lap with you, to challenge you and to be your pacesetters and grace givers. Ask them to read this book with you. It will help them to help you and also prepare them for their own bell lap someday. Their lives will be better for it and so will yours. It's a win-win.

Bucket Lists

Everyone can come up with a list of what they want to do before they kick the bucket. Doing so doesn't commit you to kicking it. List the places you want to visit, and then do it. See those childhood homes and favorite playgrounds, colleges and favorite hangouts, where you proposed (or were proposed to), where you were married, and where the children were born. Grab your picture album and someone special and visit memories one by one. List your favorite people and go see them. List your favorite foods and consume them, experience them, celebrate them. List your favorite movies and watch them again, your favorite songs and listen to them, your favorite games and play them. Make lists on tired days and check them off on energetic ones. When you reach the end, start over. I have some patients who are on their third round. There are others who only got part way through their first round, but were glad they got started early. The ones who didn't bother are just too sad to comment on.

Your times of inactivity or low energy also deserve a list. Write your life story or your memoirs; even if you don't like writing, write anyway. It is not for publishing, so don't worry about form, just pick up a journal and start. You can decide later whether to share it with someone or to burn it. Recount those pivotal, life defining, essential moments in your life. Recount your blessings and acknowledge those people who made a difference in your life and why.

If you try to make it a narrative that explains how and why you became the person you are, you may make some meaningful discoveries to both you and to others. Write love letters to your spouse and your children. Investigate your family tree, organize picture albums in a binder or online, blowup special pictures as gifts. Create a movie of you just being you, perhaps with a message to someone special. Record your voice reading a favorite children's book, gifting it to your kids and grandkids, present and/or future. When the time comes to pass the baton, you'll be ready.

This is not about getting ready to die; it is about really living instead of just being alive. I'm trying to get you running your bell lap unburdened and with as much style, meaning, and fun as possible. I know the sooner you start to run the longer it will seem and that is what matters to you and everyone else.

Got-to-do List

While you are making the "want-to-do" list, also make the "got-to-do" list and start getting to work on it. Get key documents completed and collated such as your will or Living Trust, your power of attorney for health care matters, and your power of attorney for legal matters. Make a Living Will which directs how you wish to be cared for if you are unconscious and unable to make decisions; don't leave room for your kids to argue about your wishes when you are not there to discuss them. Do estate planning, title transfers on cars and boats, and whatever. This pre-planning is one of the kindest things you can do for those you love and it lightens your load and theirs.

You can even have fun doing your will. I just redid my own. I decided to direct the first dollars of whatever is left to funding experiences. One fund is for my kids to have adventures together without spouses, one for guys with the guys, another for girls with the girls, one with spouses, and another for each grandkid to have a 1:1 adventure with my child/their parent. Relationships are precious and I want to invest in them before leaving my kids money to buy a new washing machine or barbecue. There may only be enough left for a burger and a movie, but it is the catalyst for relationships that counts.

Make lists of key people and commission the ones who will be your children's role models to fill your vacancy. Make lists of key people you rely upon and their contact information for your spouse, such as pastors, attorneys, accountants, insurance agents, various repair and maintenance people, brokers, bankers, counselors, builders, plumbers, tech gurus, doctors, and funeral directors. Then make source lists for key supplies including special foods, heating oil or gas, firewood, tires, etc. Document maintenance schedules for the car, furnace, septic system, gardens, and roof. Inventory your assets and where they are located. Even inventory your belongings—the things that matter, mementos, heirlooms, furniture or art that might be of value unknown to your spouse and kids. Then go over it all with your spouse and one of the kids. These are things you must start in the first stretch. The sooner you get them done, the sooner you can forget about them and just run. Do it now before the disease beats you up or the dragon tears you down. Lighten your load. Those trying to run weighted down are easy prey for ole fire breath.

If you are already tired, recruit someone else to do it, but get it done. Picking out a casket doesn't mean being eager to get in it. Deciding where to have your ashes spread can make for a reflective day, as can scripting a memorial service, up to and even including a message, if you like. Remember, this is just planning for a possibility, not accepting an immediate inevitability. Shuck your burdens and get ready to run.

Now is not a time to waste on maintaining the stuff of life you can live without. Get rid of what you can. Offload responsibilities that are not in the center of your passions and calling. You will surprise no one with your requests and most will bend over backwards to respond. Many friends want to help and are left waiting for the opportunity. Honor them by asking. It gives those who can't find words an opportunity to express their loving concern by helping. Give them a chance to bless you.

Making these lists and starting to check them off is really just about getting you into the first corner of your lap. Even though it may take the whole lap to check them all off, you will do better by just making the lists and getting started.

As you get into the first corner, no matter how good and meaningful your lists are, you may not be able to shake the feeling that your situation really sucks. It's okay to say it, and then move on. Don't dwell on it. Sometimes, too much energy is expended on maintaining the fiction that "everything is fine." It isn't. You need all your energy for the good stuff, not acting out the phony stuff.

Despite the loss of control of your circumstances, you can absolutely control your attitude. There's nothing that will buoy your outlook more than helping others. That's for the far corner, but first focus on your work in the near corner and some great stuff in the backstretch. I am not saying abandon your current service roles altogether, but I am trying to give you permission to focus on yourself and the hurdles before you. You will be a better servant, parent, spouse, and friend later if you do. There is some critical stuff that my patients on the track have taught me that I want to share with you. What you do with it will become an essential part of your legacy.

First Stretch Winners To-do List

- Identify those things you can control and those you cannot.
- Understand your new environment: ask your doctor for time line graphs.
- Get and understand your prognosis.
- Pay attention and walk your own walk.
- Keep your own records.
- Cut down your workload and responsibilities and delegate.
- Recruit teammates.
- Train yourself to run with both feet: hope and acceptance.
- Do your family planning.
- Make your Want-to-do and Got-to-do lists.

Chapter 5

Choosing Your Number One Goal

I t's time to get clear on your number one goal. I know you have six or twenty, but you have got to narrow it down—then keep your eyes fixed on it in every segment of your run. Otherwise, the Dragon will try to distract you and get you focusing on the wrong things.

Don't be flippant about this; I am talking about your number one goal in life. Before facing a disease and the threat of death, it may well have been about achieving things or getting stuff, goals that are suddenly losing their luster. Getting cancer can change your outlook, so give it some thought. For most people, it is to achieve and ensure the greatest number of *Symptom-Free-Days* (days free from both the symptoms of cancer and its treatment) in order to continue cherished relationships.

In order to focus in on this number one goal, there are more things that the winners must do. You need to master those things in order to come out of the near corner running hard. They won't go away until you deal with them. If left undone, they will destroy or at least shorten your backstretch where the best of the rest of your life is going to take place. You don't want to have to waste the precious backstretch on remedial unfinished near corner stuff.

Head Time and Soul Time

Before you can choose your goals, lengthen your stride, and get on with the rest of life, you had better spend some *head time* in research and some *soul time* in introspection. Head time is for the first of three things.

First, become confident in your doctors. Be certain that you can understand and communicate with them, that they take time to listen to you, and that they seem knowledgeable and decisive.

Second, get a handle on the kinds of decisions you must confront and what factors will influence your ability to make those decisions in your best interest.

Third, introspection is for identifying the adversary of your heart and soul, the Dragon. It is on the track in various disguises, but always has its claws of fear, depression, denial, and bargaining ready to latch on to you and take you out. Be proactive and start looking for those claws and get out of their reach now. Defeating the whole Dragon comes later.

Deal with those undisguised fears right in front of you that are easy to see and name by answering these questions starting right now:

Do you have the right doctor?

How do the systems of cancer clinics and hospitals, nurses and doctors really work?

What is standard therapy, alternative therapy, and what are the research options?

Are they available to you, or do you need to travel somewhere else to get them?

What does all this jargon they are using really mean?

How do you digest all this information and make decisions?

Must you just surrender your intellect and feelings to be chewed up and spit out by the medical machine?

Check Out Your Doctors

Investigate your doctor. Charm doesn't guarantee competency because quacks have plenty of it. Knowledge about the behavior and treatment of individual cancers is expanding at an extraordinary rate, so ask your oncologist how he is keeping up with the latest research. I have learned new things reading research journals before work or attending research meetings that have saved patient's lives the very next day. You want to know if your doctor goes to the yearly ASCO (American Society of Clinical Oncology) meetings or other gatherings where the latest research is discussed. Be specific. Ask where, when, and how much time he or she spends reading journals each week and which ones. Any competent, up-to-date physician will be pleased to tell you how much of his or her unpaid time is invested in study and preparation for patient care. If ongoing education in the fast-moving, ever evolving field of cancer medicine is not a priority for him/her, either find another doctor, or at least get another opinion now and then to affirm the accuracy of your treatment plan.

Second opinions are always an option, but not always necessary. If you want one and you like your physician, say you have been advised to periodically get second opinions. Then tell the new consultant upfront that you are not looking to change physicians, but you would like to review your treatment plan and get recommendations. Be aware that there are sometimes several good types of treatment, some of which may differ from yours. Analyzing and choosing between them can be difficult, but once educated, you are in a better position to ask your physician to explain whatever he recommends and be an active partner in your care.

Most cancers actually grow slowly, albeit relentlessly— although it never seems that way. When you discover it, it seems like it grew overnight when it has actually been at it for many months and probably years. So you usually have a few weeks to figure out the best doctor and the best treatment. I hope your journey starts out on the right course with the right physician, but if it doesn't, it's far better to switch even in the middle of the stream. Confidence in your doctor as an accurate source of information protects you from the fearful, often irrelevant experiences of other patients and keeps you from turning to the often misleading Internet for an answer to every question.

If you connect better with the second or third physician and he/she seems knowledgeable, just stay with them. You deserve a good fit which means comfort, confidence, and communication. You should be in control and should decide each visit whether to stay or leave. You deserve answers to your questions in a language you can understand. You are the paying customer, so keep asking until the answers make sense. You have been referred to a doctor, but that doesn't mean you are obliged to stay with them. However, they are legally obliged to stick with you forever or until they have carefully transferred your care to another doctor who is willing to accept the transfer.

All the records that have been created and accumulated about you are your property, including all office and hospital notes, all lab, x-ray, scan, and treatment records. You can request them any time and even at every visit. Many patients do. Some collect their records because they are curious, some because they travel frequently, and some because they want to consult another physician. Every doctor is obliged to provide the records whenever requested, but as it is a low tech, often low priority service, it will likely be relegated to the bottom of the to-do list of the least experienced staff member. I suggest you advise them when you will be coming to pick up the copied records and do so yourself. Decline their offer to mail the records so as to avoid the frustration of their failing to send them on time and blaming it on the mail service.

Good doctors welcome second opinions as they are always eager to improve your care. Mediocre ones resist because they are insecure and need your business, so if you encounter resistance, get your records and run to someone else. If you choose to transfer your care, in addition to getting your records, ask the physician you are leaving to kindly write the new physician a transfer letter describing his assessment of you and the behavior of your unique cancer situation.

Transferring care is very doable at any point in your care, but the longer you have been with a physician, the more information that physician and his office staff have of you and your disease that is not in print. Because you would rather not transfer care later, you should get your due diligence done early. Size your physicians up. Take your family along. Ask friends and nurses all about them. You should be comfortable asking your physician any question and be confident that he is shooting straight with you on the answers. He should be willing to give you all the time you need and you should be able to get prompt responses from the office staff when you have questions or concerns. A critical review early on can save time and disappointment later.

They get paid for the amount of time they spend with you on medical issues and for the complexities of your problems, but not for socializing and often not for counseling. You will need to find care for your heart, soul, and all Dragon issues elsewhere, but when it comes to medical issues don't let them cut you off and don't waste their time with chit chat.

What You Need to Know About Cancer Clinics

There are some things you need to know about doctors and their offices that will enable you to help them help you. Get to know key nurses and receptionist by their first names and ask for them by name whenever possible. It is huge. Write them down or have your teammate do it on the first visit and learn them. It establishes a connection which can make a difference when you call for assistance. Every office is swamped with complex people with complex problems. If you make that simple connection, they will subliminally pay more attention to you and remember more about your problems which can make a big difference when you call for help.

If you have a need, the earlier in the day and in the week that you call, the more resources and flexibility they will have to assist with your problem, and the less likely you will end up in a tedious

Emergency Waiting Room just to see an unfamiliar physician. Procrastinating until the end of the day, the end of the week, or until after hours will only reward you with frustration and perhaps a new on-call doctor, both of which increase your chances of being hospitalized.

Most doctors are compassionate and well-trained, but they are all human. The good ones are often in high demand, consequently overcommitted and behind schedule. They are also often dealing with multiple patients simultaneously. If you choose appointments earlier in the morning or right after lunch you will get a less harried doctor with more mental energy he can focus on you.

Go to appointments prepared with a written list of prioritized observations and problems.

You will get better care if you can give your doctor a written list of all your questions as soon as he comes into the room. That will enable him to prioritize the time he will spend with you and give the most important issues the most time. I have been astonished by patients who are socially engaging and leisurely wander through minor issues only to pop their most important question last when I am out of time and halfway out the door.

A written list also lets the doctor know that what you have given him has not only been carefully thought-out in advance, but that you are also respectful of him and his schedule. Making the list helps you because it requires you to analyze your experiences and collect your thoughts. If you have symptoms, write them down. Just the process of making the written list will surprise you with new discoveries—things you have forgotten or associations you have overlooked before. Help your doctor help you—do you part.

If medications bother you, record how and when. If you have pains, keep a record of where they are and scale their severity 1-10. Do this throughout the day. Record how well the medicines work and how long. That may seem like too much of a bother, but if you have serious pain and you want effective medications with the least side effects, then get serious about describing it to your doctor. Do the same for other symptoms like nausea, shortness of breath, dizziness, and painful urination.

When listening to a physician answer your questions, don't rely on your memory. Have a family member or friend along to take notes, or take a tape recorder, or both.

Medicare and other insurance companies reimburse doctors for the amount of time they spend with patients and the complexity of their problems. The amount of time allotted and reimbursed is limited and often inadequate. Therefore, if you come with a well-thought-out and prioritized list of problems and address them directly, you are more likely to get enough of his time to deal with them. Enjoy the interpersonal, relationship building stuff, but save it for the end of the visit when you're sure there is time to spare. When your doctor takes the time to really listen to you, tell him how grateful you are. Remember, insurance companies pay doctors to treat your disease not to teach you how to live. You need to be real clear about what is important to you and convey that to him. His primary focus is going to be on length of life, not what you do with it.

A Word of Caution about Physicians

You need to be aware of what influences physicians. If you understand the economic, medical-legal, insurance reimbursement, and time utilization forces that shape physician behavior, it will change your questioning and decision-making process. One physician told me that he considered every patient a potential lawsuit waiting to happen. So the more anxious, critical or confrontational a patient is, the more tests and consultations a doctor will order, both to answer patient's concerns, but also to protect themselves in the event of a lawsuit.

Ordering tests is very easy for physicians and costs them nothing, but testing does consume your time and your money. Sometimes, tests are done more frequently than is really necessary for decision making just as a matter of routine or to protect a nervous patient or doctor. If you are someone who has the time and money to spare and wants lots of extra information, then extra tests may be perfect for you.

There is, however, a risk that an unnecessary test will uncover a slight abnormality that may be irrelevant, but will cause more anxiety and lead to even further tests. I encourage patients to ask their doctors what they expect to be learned from a given blood test, x-ray or scan and how it will affect their treatment decisions. Faced with that question, physicians are less likely to order tests as a matter of routine or just to assuage your anxiety or theirs. If you are not anxious, they will be less anxious. That is to your advantage.

Financial Toxicity Is Associated with Adverse Outcomes

The cost of cancer care has spiraled upwards. The stress it can cause can adversely affect quality of life, the tolerance of therapy, and the length of life itself. Doctors are often unaware of the actual costs of the care they prescribe and even less aware of your ability to embrace those costs. The Hippocratic Oath does not commission them to be very interested in discussing either one, but they will if you initiate the discussion.

The current average chemotherapy cost per month is estimated at $10,000. Insurance co-pays are rising and the cost of some of the newest and least toxic biologic or oral chemotherapies are often not covered. A study of insured cancer patients at an academic medical center found, "72% of patients applied for copayment assistance, 42% found their cancer treatment a significant or catastrophic burden, and 46% stinted on food and clothing to pay for their medications...Adherence was compromised in 63% and 24% avoided taking drugs altogether." (Please be aware that the results of any treatment program are dependent on a patient receiving at least 80% of the prescribed dose on time.) A separate study in the state of Washington showed that "cancer patients had a 2.65% times greater risk of bankruptcy compared to the general population."[10]

Many patients intend to talk to their physicians about costs, but only a fraction do. However, those who did frequently had the cost of their care reduced, and 75 percent of the time it was possible without changing treatment. Have that talk each time treatment changes. There may come a time when the possible benefits of treatment are outweighed by exorbitant costs and that information can be critical in making the best decision for you and your family.

What Is Standard Therapy?

Have a conversation with your physician about "standard therapy," which is defined as a time-tested regimen, a combination of medicines given in a particular sequence over a particular time period for a particular cancer that over the years has yielded the best responses for a large heterogeneous group of patients. In order to have reached this status, a regimen has had to be created and tested over a period of time and the results observed for at least five years or more. There are two potential drawbacks to such standard therapy.

The first occurs if the unique characteristics of your disease do not match the majority of patients studied, in which case it is unwise to assume that the study results of the standard therapy will reliably apply to your special situation. For example, breast cancer is like apples; not everyone is the same. Some apples are red, others yellow or green, some sweet others tart, and recipes for pies vary. Standard regimens/recipes for breast cancer are perfect for some, but not all.

The second is that any new effective drugs or combination of drugs that has been discovered in the last five years will not yet be part of the good old standard therapy. While many times standard therapy is precisely what you need, it is worth asking your physician if there are other therapies or newer drugs that might better suit your unique situation that are worth considering. Standard therapy is an easy and safe recommendation for a physician who is anxious about lawsuits. Expressing interest in other therapies invites him to treat you as a unique individual rather than as a category.

Research Options

Proffered questions about other therapies may also open the door to discussing various research options. If he doesn't know of any, you may want another opinion, not because you necessarily want to be on a study, but because you want a doctor who is at least familiar with the cutting edge of knowledge and research.

Participating in a research study often means being randomized by the flip of a coin to taking a standard therapy or one of new design: old drugs in a new combination or new drugs. New is not always better, hence the reason for the study, so it is worth asking the physician which arm of the study he favors. He should know the results of the latest research which were the basis for designing the newest study. If he doesn't have an opinion about which arm he would choose for himself, then going on the study is a fine option.

If, however, he has a reason to believe one arm of the study is better than another for your unique situation, then it is worth seriously considering taking the treatment in that arm, but off study instead of going on the study even if it is not the standard therapy. His recommendation may well become the new standard when the results of the study are analyzed five to ten years down the road. Of course, by then it might be too late for you, if you haven't gambled on your physician's best hunch. Sometimes, new studies are done just to confirm what we are pretty sure we already know. Unless you ask your doctor, he probably won't tell you which arm of the study he favors, so ask her/him.

Alternative Therapy

Some individuals have a distrust of doctors. Sometimes this is well justified and other times it is inherited. There are some terrible doctors out there and even good ones can make mistakes. Listening to those who have bad stories, it is easy to understand where their feelings come from and why they have turned away from traditional medicine. Other individuals are disappointed when their doctors and their therapies don't offer enough promise, but have potential serious side effects. Both groups can launch out on an odyssey to find an alternative therapy.

If you are one of these, beware of the siren song on the Internet or of friends extolling the miraculous responses, maybe even cures, to alternative therapies. When such extraordinary benefits are claimed and often with little toxicity, they can pique anyone's curiosity, especially when labeled "natural." Some are indeed harmless and only separate you from your money, but others can dissuade you from taking truly effective conventional treatment or worse yet may render traditional treatments ineffective or even more toxic. So, beware of a cocktail of alternative therapies if they have not been carefully studied in randomized controlled trials alone or in combination with the traditional therapies you choose. Some, such as laetrile and vitamin C have been studied in such a fashion and been found to be worthless. Another, coffee enemas, while unstudied and unproven, will, as one patient put it, leave you "clean as a whistle and high as a kite."

The Federal Trade Commission is using education and enforcement to guard the vulnerable from the con artists. It maintains a website, www.ftc.gov. I would encourage you to check out. It cautions people to be skeptical, helping them to sort truth from fiction, as some therapies are just plain scams. It provides a few useful tips similar to what I've been telling people for thirty years, such as to be leery of any product that asserts it works for all cancers and all people. Every cancer is different. Extensive studies show that the same type of cancer in different individuals may have varied responses to the same treatment.

A product labeled "natural" does not guarantee it is either effective or safe. It doesn't even mean that it is natural. It does mean that it has not been evaluated or tested for safety by the Federal Drug Administration (FDA). Testimonies may seem heartfelt and honest and still be totally false. Personal stories from sincere people are often unintentionally unreliable and inaccurate. In particular, beware of endorsements by celebrities.

Technical jargon does not mean it is scientific or effective even though it sounds impressive. A money back guarantee is no substitute for scientific evidence. Beware of meaningless terms such as all natural, antioxidant rich, clinically proven, anti-aging, and other vague, but seductive claims.

Beware of adulterated products that can be obtained over-the-counter, hand-to-hand, or through the mail. The FDA has withdrawn over 140 products that were laced with undisclosed pharmaceutical ingredients. Perhaps the most shameful example was PG-SPES, a supplement easily obtainable without a prescription, which was heavily promoted to treat prostate cancer. The stuff actually did lower prostatic specific antigen (PSA) levels, a standard test used to monitor prostate cancer therapy, but not because of its eight mysterious Chinese herbs, but rather because it was laced with potent pharmaceuticals: an estrogen (diethylstilbestrol), along with an anticoagulant (warfarin) and a nonsteroidal anti-inflammatory drug (indomethacin) all of which have potentially dangerous side effects in some individuals.[11] Supplements are not evaluated by the FDA and therefore do not offer the protection of prescription medications.

Con Artist Scam Indicators

- Product is asserted to work for:

  Many or all cancers

  Many or all people

  Several diseases of different origins
- Products labeled as "natural, anti-oxidant, or anti-aging"
- Personal testimonials – especially from celebrities
- Impressive technical jargon, including "clinically proven"
- Money back guarantee

Chapter 6

Near Corner Reevaluation

I am speaking to three groups of people now: those who might be cured already, those who will take a limited course of treatment giving them a shot at cure, and those who are incurable and desperately seeking a remission knowing full well there will be some kind of treatment on and off for the rest of their lives. Much of this chapter is most urgent for the latter group who already hear the Dragon whispering, but every bit of it is just as critical for the first two groups. The Dragon will be waiting for them as soon as they finish their treatment and start the *long wait* wondering, "Am I really cured?" It is a question that no doctor can answer and one that the Dragon can use to mess with their heads forever. So, all three groups had best pay attention now or dance with the Dragon later.

To get into the near corner, all groups have started some form of therapy: surgery, radiation or chemo. You have discovered what is involved and tasted your first side effects. You are probably relaxing a bit having made your first big decisions and begun an attack on the cancer. While you are breathing a little easier, it is time to re-examine the assumptions that guided your decisions and what subliminal things influenced them. All of you are going to have more decisions ahead – especially every time there is a new ache or pain, lump or bump or change in therapy. Learn now and you will be better prepared for the next decision – and there is always another decision.

After the opening campaign in any war when the scope of the conflict is emerging, a good general will reevaluate their initial assumptions that led to their battle plan and decide if they were accurate then and are they still accurate now. Were they fooled and if so, how? You need to do the same as the character of the disease and the impact of therapy on stamina and lifestyle emerge. Then use what you learn to form your next decision.

World War II was about so much more than what was obviously going on in the blatant conflict. It was also about trench foot, dysentery, frostbite, supply lines, fear, fitness, and the Holocaust. When you're a few months into your cancer battle, you may discover that cancer treatment affects your life in more ways than you had imagined, especially the fatigue and other toxicities that are cumulative over time. It's time to reconcile the reality of treatment with one's assumptions and expectations—not necessarily to abandon it, but to change those things under your control.

Preview Far Corner Rounding Decisions

It may be possible to put even an incurable cancer into remission a few times and in some cases, like breast cancer, several times. Every time the disease progresses, even though the finish line is not in view, the same kind of challenging decisions must be made. Each one is a prelude to those critical ones in the far corner—the corner no one likes to think about especially now. However, if you practice thinking these decisions through with each progression, you will be prepared when you find yourself suddenly coming into or out of that corner. That is where many stumble. The belief that you will never progress is fine, but it will not protect you from the Dragon who will haunt you anyway with the risk that you might. Don't kid yourself. Where there is risk the Dragon will exploit it. Preparing is like putting on a Kevlar vest that the Dragon cannot penetrate.

If you ponder these issues early, you will be ready because when the time comes it is often a surprise. The sooner you think it through, the sooner you protect the quality of the rest of your life. The Dragon will want to use it, like every other unknown, as a weapon to spoil your joy. So, let's review disease progression decision issues, then set that tough subject aside, and return to running the near corner and looking forward to a long, fun, and meaningful backstretch.

If the disease progresses requiring a change in therapy, the risks, expectations, and prognosis are often not readdressed by the physician with the same diligence as they did early on. Many patients really don't want to know. They would rather live with outdated information than have to deal with new unfavorable information.

Beware: Unexamined assumptions can cause misinformed decisions.

A traditional attitude of many people is that the ends must justify the means. You need to know that cancers progress by outsmarting the original therapies which were often chosen both because they were best but also because they were the least toxic. Hence, what is left are the treatments that are less effective and more toxic. In addition, everyone at this stage will be more vulnerable to the toxicities because they are already weakened by the cumulative effect of growing cancer, and the now just abandoned ineffective treatment.

The possibility of increased toxicity may get little discussion or may be sanitized by the physician if he thinks there is no other choice. However, there is always another positive choice and you're the only one who can make it. Bravely consider not taking the new therapy. Perhaps, the ends don't justify the means. Perhaps, the ends have no chance of being what you hope for. You need to know. Perhaps, your life would be better without it. In such a situation, choosing not to take it is a positive choice, a wise and courageous choice—the right choice.

What matters to most people is Real Survival, which is the Quality of life expressed as a percent of normal, multiplied times the duration of life measured in days.

Clearly, if the quality of days alive is so lousy that you can't enjoy it as you wish, then having more of it is less valuable than high quality time for fewer days. The unintended, seldom discussed reality is that most patients assume any treatment is going to lengthen their overall lifetime, Real Survival. That is patently false for most third or fourth-line treatments.

You must insist on an accurate assessment of what you can personally expect for your exact condition in terms of outcome and toxicity in order to make your best decision. Only the wisdom of your physician can give you this, not the literature or the internet. Physicians are often afraid of hurting your feelings with the truth. If you want it, ask for it straight up.

Even less often discussed is how expectations have changed. After a relapse, the chance of long-term, meaningful, symptom-free remission will have declined, sometimes dramatically. Again, it depends upon the type, grade, stage, and the *degree of progression*. There needs to be careful discussion, so that you can be sure the ends proffered really justify the means.

An assertion that a treatment is "new" can create unjustified expectations, so ask the hard questions. Be aware that reported response rates (RR) alone are often misleading unless the responses are long-lasting, expressed in terms of prolonged response duration (MDR: median duration of remission), and overall survival (OS). Small or uncertain chances of response are meaningless in the face of toxicities that are 100 percent guaranteed and would better be avoided.

Witch Doctors and Which Medicines

In 2009, my son Trevor and I were working in a destitute refugee squatter's village in Zambia near the border of the embattled Congo. Our goal was to figure out how to improve the health education of children in a mission school in hopes of both affecting their generation, but also of creating an inroad through the kids' literacy to their illiterate parents. We had a chance to talk with a pastor and a healthcare worker about the response of these people to the threat of death from AIDS, TB or malaria. We wondered how they coped with approaching death without the hopes or the false hopes of modern medical technology.

We wondered if we would discover an aboriginal tradition of wisdom, grace, and destiny as Murray Trelease had found with the coastal Natives of British Columbia. We didn't. Instead, we heard stories of the same disabling fear of death that we see in the West, only in Zambia it drove them to witch doctors, who skillfully manipulated their fears to separate them from their money and meager possessions. A pattern of expensive mumbo jumbo witchcraft, hope, anxiety, failure to improve, and despair was repeated until their resources were exhausted or their lives lost. The Dragon is clearly active there in a different culture, but using the same tactics of fear and manipulation.

We in the West are haunted by the same Dragon. Here only a few cast their lives at the feet of witch doctors, just an occasional quack. Instead, more often we cast our hopes at the altar of "which medicine" until we are ensnared in the same exhausted bodies, finances, and hopes until we give up and die. We do have some wonderful medicines, but there comes a time when even those no longer work and your best choice is to stop trying new ones.

Length and quality of survival does depend on which doctor you choose, but it also depends on which hopes you choose to stake your life on.

Our society's health care system will not help you navigate your way through the really tough health/soul care decisions. It has no weapons to fight the Dragon. You need to do your homework while you are able, so you will be ready to make decisions in your own best interest if that time comes, as it will for many. There is a point at which less is more and you need to be prepared to find it. Start imagining yourself in that situation now and how you will make such a decision. Remember, one face of cowardice is postponing a decision until it is no longer relevant.

Don't put this book down if you think there is too much emphasis on the fourth quarter, endgame, home stretch, and finish line stuff. I'm convinced that your whole game, your whole bell lap, your whole fight with cancer will go better and be more successful if you start thinking about and even preparing for the home stretch right now, which seldom means you plan to get there very soon. I've watched a lot of people do it both ways. It is not how you start that counts, but how you finish.

You never need lose to cancer, even if it takes your life. You can beat cancer every time by how you live, why you live, and in the manner in which you live.[10]

Homestretch Holiday Option

You are probably thinking this is a ridiculous topic and inappropriate, even depressing, especially where you are at right now. That is both true and false. You are not there now and that is why it won't be depressing now, sobering maybe but empowering. Everything you think about now and bring under your control takes away from the Dragon's ammunition to use to scare and manipulate you from here on out. The more you know the more control you have, the less uncertainty and the more peace.

If any of this gets too heavy, skip ahead for now, but come back later. This is important stuff you don't want to miss.

Cancer rarely takes a life suddenly, so most everyone who is not in denial will get a homestretch. No one looks forward to it, but if run well, it can be an extraordinary time that no one would want to miss. You can get up from the table after the main course, but why skip dessert if you don't have to.

Hopefully, the homestretch is a long way off, but even so it will be better run with preparation. It will pose challenging questions and the Dragon will be there messing with your head. You had best start thinking about them now. If you do, your readiness will afford you a measure of peace and grace for the rest of your run. If you consider how to make the tough homestretch decisions now, it will actually help you make other pesky ones in the interim. Those in denial will likely blow by this section.

If the disease relapses a second time and is found to be growing despite a second course of treatment or combination of drugs, it means for most that the homestretch is not far off. With the exception of breast cancer and very few others, a third or fourth type of treatment is unlikely to significantly lengthen your life, but you are likely to be offered it anyway because many doctors don't know what else to do.

So you must ask,
"What is the average prolongation of survival for an
average patient with my stage of my disease
with the treatment proposed?"

Get ready for all kinds of hedging. The precise information you need is hard to come by. The doctor usually can't just look it up. He can certainly give you his best educated estimate, though. There are different types and grades of cancer and there are exceptions to what I'm going to say next, but they are only exceptions. If you have metastatic cancer that has failed at least one treatment regimen and is therefore usually incurable, expect his answer about the prolongation of survival by new treatment to be measured in weeks to months. Failing one regimen usually means incurability and failing two means chances of much further benefit from any treatment are usually small.

It was 2010 when I first wrote that paragraph and now an addendum is in order. Immunotherapy is coming of age and will certainly improve in years to come. It is different in mechanisms of action and side effects but sadly as yet only works in a select few but ever growing number of cancers and patients

In some cancers genetic changes can be detected and matched to specific therapies targeting molecules inside and on the surface of the tumor cells. Examples include the immune check point inhibitors that enable immune T lymphocytes to attack the tumor. And others include engineered antibodies directed at specific sites uniquely found on the cancer cells. The two-strikes-and- you-are-out rule applies to chemotherapies not these targeted therapies.

Breast cancer, lymphomas, and a very few others are exceptions to this rule, but the same issues will arise eventually for them as well, so always ask the question. The truth is often so shocking that physicians won't offer it unless you ask, but you need to know. Both the length and the quality of the time you have left hinges upon your next decision and may both be longer and better if you say no to another treatment. You can only do that if you have all the available information.

At this point, be especially wary of the lure of experimental therapies and apply the same rigid questioning. I have been asked, "What is the best way to press the doctor for truthful but negative information?" Sometimes, there exists a willful bias towards hope in the physician. He will feel it and squirm and not give the raw truth to you unless you ask. Simply say, "Doc, I need to know the worst case. Give it to me straight."

Beware if the word "maybe" is ever used.
Make certain to get what is meant clearly defined.
Otherwise, your hopeful heart is likely to erroneously
ascribe all kinds of unrealistic expectations to the word.

Here is why this is so important. Frequently, when I have this conversation with a patient who has failed two chemotherapy regimens, their average survival is only three to nine months. Often, the best treatment option could only prolong their life an average of a few weeks or a few months—or not at all. We know that when there are three, six, or nine months left, the last month will be unpleasant, and most likely in bed. The one to two months before that will likely be problematic, and at least mediocre, with poor appetite, energy, and ambition compelling most to stay near home and the clinic. However, the first few months are going to be the very best and will be the last good months remaining for good times, celebration, and travel. They may not be as good as a patient would like, but they will be the best that is left.

The only way for the patient to get any better at this point is to stop treatment and thereby avoid the side effects, as well as tests and clinic visits, which are no longer necessary. Most who stop treatment will start feeling somewhat or occasionally a lot better for a while, as the cumulative bad effects from previous treatment wear off. This holiday will last until the inevitable cancer symptoms recur, usually weeks to months down the road.

The only situation in which patients miss out on this holiday is when they don't quit soon enough and keep hopping only on their right foot—hope. Choosing to drag their left foot—acceptance, they will endure ineffective treatment and postpone stopping until they are actively dying with all kinds of symptoms from the cancer and have no other choice. Most good doctors can sense when a treatment is no longer working, but if patients are feeling okay, they don't want to hear the bad news. Many doctors delay the bad news and continue worthless therapy to offer hope, albeit false hope, until the patient has more symptoms and their dying body tells them the truth, invariably too late. It is easier for a patient to hear the word "hopeless" from a doctor when their body is already feeling terrible, but at that point they have missed their holiday off treatment and everything they could have done with it. It can be such a precious time. Don't miss it.

Near Corner Reevaluation

- Go to appointments prepared with a written list of prioritized observations and problems.

- What matters to most people is Real Survival, which is the quality of life free of symptoms of treatment and cancer expressed as a percent of normal multiplied by the duration of life measured in days.

- quality of life expressed as a percent of normal, multiplied times the duration of life measured in days.

- You must insist on an accurate assessment of what you can personally expect for your exact condition in terms of outcome and toxicity in order to make your best decision.

- Length and quality of survival does depend on which doctor you choose, but it also depends on which hopes you choose to stake your life on.

- Beware if the word "maybe" is ever used. Make certain to get what is meant clearly defined.

Chapter 7

Decisions and How to Make Them

When it seems that cancer is taking everything from you, you still have choices to make: critical decisions that will ultimately determine the length and quality of your life. You better make them well. You will need to make them again and again every time there is a change in disease behavior or treatment. Therefore, it is essential to understand the decision-making process.

It must be a team process with the doctor. He may have tunnel vision focused on the biologic necessities and consequences of any treatment decision. He/she will gather all the information from your exam and tests, but the right and best decisions will only be possible with your active participation. The physician will attempt to figure it all out, but will be limited by the information and guidance you provide. There are no single right answers. You need to integrate your life necessities with his treatment possibilities. When cancer cannot be cured and becomes chronic and ultimately life-threatening, the personal, social, and spiritual arenas of life become ever more important, and only you can identify them and put them in the treatment decision equation.

However, as the specter of advancing disease consumes ever more attention, these are often undervalued or overlooked by the doctors unless you make a point of prioritizing them. If you have not made a point of figuring out what is of greatest meaning and importance to you between relationships, avocations, work, and spiritual journey, and communicate it repeatedly to your physician, you will be treated like an automaton characterized by laboratory data and physical exam findings. We are talking about it all now so you can figure it out before you are faced with critical decisions. Cancer just happens to some people who don't think ahead. Don't be one of them.

At the outset, meaning, purpose, and priority are almost universally condensed into, "Keep me alive, Doc." But the further you get in your cancer experience and the further you get on your bell lap, the more other priorities will become apparent and need expression. Treatment should not be "one-size-fits-all," but it will become so unless you are continuously and actively involved.

Critical Decision Pathway

Whether you choose to relinquish decision-making entirely to your physician, you choose to be intimately involved, or you choose to involve God, it is useful to understand the human decision-making process.

Neuroscientists have learned that there is an anatomic area of the brain that is absolutely necessary for decision-making called the prefrontal cortex. It functions like a workbench where we place all the components of the problem that needs solving. There we sort them out, prioritize them, and craft a solution. It is functionally called our "working memory." The more clutter that is placed on the bench, the slower the decision-making process and the more likely an irrelevant decision will be reached.

Each individual will be faced with a complex array of new and ever-changing information which must be either selected and integrated or discarded from the bench. Few decisions in cancer are urgent (remember that), although they all feel emergent. However, if you put off making decisions too long, you risk overloading your workbench and your decision-making circuitry, which may lead ultimately to poor decisions. So, be disciplined and expeditious now to avoid ever having to be frantic later.

More important than speed in decision making is identifying and focusing on critical pieces of information and goals.

Only after distinguishing between what is possible, what is probable, and what is hoped for should you then decide on a course of action. You don't ever need to let go of what is hoped for, but you must not let it blind you. Walk through your decisions with both shoes on.

When a pilot loses all the hydraulics that control the ailerons, wing flaps, and rudder that steer and fly the plane, critical decisions need to be made as to how to get the plane on the ground safely. There are dozens of dials reading out bits of information in front of him and hysteria in the cabin behind him. Likewise, a scrambling NFL quarterback with eyes scanning down field as the pocket collapses around him must deal with a similar information overload as he searches for a receiver. Both pilot and quarterback must follow a critical decision pathway even though both situations are fluid with parameters changing moment by moment in the air or on the playing field.

There are people who study these decisions and write about them such as, Jonah Lehrer, in *How We Decide*. They examine not just what the right decisions are, but how they are made, which techniques make the difference between a safe landing and catastrophe, between getting sacked and tossing a game-winning pass. They found that stellar pilots and winning quarterbacks are able to deal selectively despite emotional overload and the overwhelming amount of changing information by focusing on the most important pieces of data. "They were always thinking about what they should think about, which let them minimize potential distractions." For instance, when pilot Al Haynes' DC 10 was disabled after flying into a flock of geese, he realized that he could not steer; he had no rudder or flap control. He only had control of the throttle levers to produce variable thrust in the remaining two engines. Everything else in the cockpit was virtually useless, so he immediately zeroed in on the possibility of steering with his engines. [12]

It is equally important for the cancer patient to prioritize bits of information and focus their thoughts. You must make a conscious effort to clear the clutter off your working memory workbench. That means discarding every bit of biologic information, every symptom, and every emotionally charged issue which doesn't bear directly on the next decision at hand. You also need to suspend your work/play schedule and unload to others as many other decision-making responsibilities in the rest of your life as possible until your health decisions are made. You can pick those other decisions back up later, but for now clear your bench. Then ask your doctor what the key issues are and ignore the rest at least temporarily. When he tells you he is not concerned about a little pain here or there, a sneeze or gas pains in your belly or whatever, then let them go. Report everything and then discard as much as you can.

Focus, focus, focus! Prioritize, prioritize, and prioritize! It is uniquely human, but still difficult, to transcend feelings and instincts in order to drill down on the facts, weigh the pros and cons, and make critical decisions.

Beware of the emotional brain which is quick to make decisions. It doesn't need all the information and it can't be bothered with deliberation and logic. That is exactly where the Dragon wants to take you. Once the emotional brain is engaged, it clambers to take control of decision-making and is resistant to considering facts. It is as if there is an emotional threshold which, once reached, abandons all reason. Emotions are important but the Dragon will rile them up. Honor them, they are real, but reign them in for decision-making.

**You need to look for and avoid emotional issues
that can preload the brain with emotional heat.**

You need to know where the Dragon lives so you can be on your guard. Pondering fearful or negative thoughts, experiencing interpersonal disharmony, losing sleep, lacking emotional support, struggling with stress at work or at home all preload our emotional brain, making it difficult to make cool and calculated decisions. If you can refocus your thoughts, avoid conflict, unload some stressful responsibilities, get your sleep (take a sleep aid if you need it), then you will be better able to focus, prioritize, and make critical pathway decisions.

Loss Aversion

We are not just machines that coldly process information. We are driven by emotion in ways we often don't even recognize. Loss aversion was first described in the 1970s by Kahneman and Trevsky and again by Jonan Lehrer. It occurs when an individual has to choose in the midst of uncertainty between two or more alternatives that bear significantly different risks, rewards, and emotional impacts. This comes into play in game shows like "Let's Make a Deal," on Wall Street, and in treatment decisions on the cancer ward. This occurs when a patient doesn't carefully evaluate all of the information necessary to calculate the probabilities in order to make a rational decision. Instead, they use "emotional instincts and mental shortcuts" that skip an analysis altogether. The fear of losing your life can be so high that it can compel you to choose a treatment which has a small likelihood of benefit. This is another place the Dragon lives.

Loss Aversion is an innate behavioral flaw that everyone who is in touch with their emotions experiences. It has been widely studied in many arenas of human endeavor, from economics to medicine. It can apply directly to your treatment decisions and the unfortunate consequences can be huge. This simple flaw in the emotional brain can cause you to make irrational decisions to choose treatments of low efficacy and high toxicity in order to save your life, even though the treatment is more likely to lessen the number of your symptom-free days. It can even shorten your life! Unless you have already experienced significant drug toxicity (and I hope you haven't), the gain in avoiding it (which is now more likely) appears too small compared to the fear of losing your life. The Dragon manipulates your emotions so your brain cannot evaluate the facts.

There is only one way to avoid falling into the loss aversion trap: know about it and watch out for it.

I saw this happen repeatedly in the setting of relapsing life-threatening cancer which had failed primary and secondary therapy. Losing hope and fearing loss of life, individuals would choose high risk "rescue" chemotherapy without giving it much thought. They often failed to question the doctor carefully about the chances of benefit or precisely what the benefit would really look like. Neither did they question what the new toxicities might be, or whether they might be worse because many of their cancer-injured organs were not working as well as they used to.

Patients seldom asked what life would be like if this treatment were not taken, falsely assuming it would be worse than taking the treatment. As a result, the busy physician often does not answer the questions that were never asked and proceeds with the high-risk therapy, which more often harms than helps. Sometimes patients don't ask the questions because they don't want to hear the answers, hopping on the right foot with hope and ignoring the left foot of acceptance. The Dragon has taken another prisoner with fear.

Every patient whose cancer has become incurable will reach a point when the best treatments are no longer effective. There comes a time when the best therapies have been used and only the mediocre ones remain. This is when decision-making gets really difficult and the loss aversion phenomena can come into play. The physician will speak of the medicine that "we can try." He may not be able to state what the chances of response are, because there is simply insufficient data available on using this medicine in patients like you for whom other treatments X, Y, and Z have been tried and abandoned due to failure. He may estimate that there will be a response rate to the new medicine in the 5, 10 or even 15 percent range. Of note is that the physician often will not say what the quality or duration of the response might be or how he expects you to feel during or after the treatment. He will often not elaborate on the side effects and seldom states the inverse; there is an 85-95 percent certainty of no response, no benefit, and a 100 percent chance of side effects.

At this point, either something the physician has said or the patient's own innate wishful thinking has conjured up the optimistic possibility of a great treatment response or possibly even a cure. A false image of a return to healthy functioning and the reappearance of the patient's pre-cancer lifestyle and dreams become a reference point and the potential gain against which all must be measured. Therefore, not to accept the treatment offered would be to lose all of that, albeit total fantasy. Loss aversion thinking can dominate the prefrontal cortex workbench.

Individuals will take extraordinary risks to avoid losing a dream, including one that is a complete misconception. Their emotions sabotage reason and their lack of accurate information sidesteps their intellect. However, now there is the compounding effect of toxicities of the chemotherapy that doesn't work in addition to the malicious effect of a growing tumor guaranteeing loss of symptom-free days.

Loss of Negative Bias Protection

Hasty emotional loss aversion decisions preclude the operation of another potentially helpful inherent human phenomenon, "negative bias," which means that we are innately more motivated by the risk of bad things than we are the lure of good things. Had the relapsing patient not been frightened into loss aversion behavior and taken the time to learn how toxic the proposed bailout therapy was, they would have realized they were about to lose the best days of the rest of their lives, and subsequently would have made a different decision.

Part of the problem is created by the way physicians speak. They know how important it is to keep hope alive, hence, they speak with a hopeful bias. The pleading eyes of their patients have taught them that when hope for medical treatment dies, they are in for a sad, often long and emotionally wrenching conversation. Sometimes, physicians are short on time, short on compassion, or emotionally tapped out, thus they focus on a thin thread of hope in a new treatment rather than a candid discussion of its risks and benefits. Unfortunately, these last-ditch treatments usually have little or no chance of working for very long. That is not the way it's supposed to be, but physicians are human and it happens.

Sadly, for some physicians it can be more sinister. The thread of hope they offer sometimes fuels their personal research by getting patients onto a clinical trial, or pads their wallets by keeping patients on expensive treatments. There are not many physicians like this, but there are some. One does well to steer clear of them, or at least be aware of such potential biases that can affect even the most virtuous physician at least subconsciously.

Rational Choice Theory

"Rational Choice Theory assumes that people make decisions by multiplying the probability of getting what they want by the amount of pleasure (utility) that getting it will bring."[13] This presupposes that one really knows what he/she wants and can reliably extract the probability of getting it from their doctor. If you can't communicate realistic goals, he has no chance of giving you realistic probabilities. Only you can figure this out and tell him.

Many people haven't really resolved what is most important and possible: the product of hoping and accepting. Even if they have, they often lack the eloquence to express it or the courage to insist their physician provide a fair estimate of achieving it with any treatment program. You must have this figured out by the end of the backstretch and, of course, you don't really know when that is; so get on with it. Peace will follow.

A study of cancer patients with less than four months to live revealed that in less than one third of the patients did a doctor ask, "What are your fears, goals, and priorities when your time is short? What outcome for you would be unacceptable?" So, if you can't count on the doctor to ask, you have to ask yourself. This is huge. Studies also show that those who have this conversation suffer less, stop chemotherapy, accept Hospice sooner, spend less time in the hospital, and in the case of lung cancer, live 25 percent longer![14]

Compromised communications with physicians can have both a gender and generational component. More women than men have not found their voice or the empowerment to use it, either out of temerity, misguided respect, or fear. In any case, silence does not serve them well. Older patients belong to a generation that was conditioned to never question the doctor, believing he is the expert and is therefore always right. Often, they are just not prepared. If you are one of these, take an assertive husband or daughter with you.

Our loss aversion proclivity can sabotage this process on two levels. We fear losing dreams and hopes, so we choose not to ask the tough questions that could confront us with the stress of needing to make tough decisions. We also fear losing our lives, hopes, and fantasies so we opt for therapies with lousy toxic/ therapeutic ratios simply because we don't know any better and are afraid to find out. Chalk another one up for the Dragon! Defeat it by finding other hopes and dreams that cancer and death cannot gnash.

It's like a batter at the plate with a three and two count taking a wild swing at a pitch that is way outside the strike zone in the hopes of scoring a home run. If he had only let it go by, he would have at least walked to first base. If a cancer patient will let the futile therapy pass by, they would at least be toxicity free on first base. One has to drive down hard on what really matters and focus on both sides of the treatment decision. You need to know what the chances are that the new treatment will actually deliver on your hopes, and recognize there is a chance that more treatment will take away something you could already have, i.e., time without treatment side effects.

Reversible Decisions Are the Safest

When you are scared, it is easy to decide to do something, only to discover later that it was worse than doing nothing at all.

It is exceedingly rare in cancer that anything must be done in a hurry. Even aggressive cancers grow slowly, although relentlessly, and are unlikely to get you into more trouble overnight or over the next week. Choosing not to do something like a new treatment is a reversible decision that enables you to ponder and pray about it for a while. You can always change your mind to take it, but once it is in your veins, it's too late.

The decision not to take a treatment or to discontinue treatment altogether, is one of the most important, liberating, and courageous decisions you will ever have the opportunity to make. Family members can make it even harder, especially if they have been protected or kept in the dark about your status and experiences. Be vulnerable all along the way and share everything with them so they can be in the same place you are when the time for tough decisions comes. It helps them process it all, support you, appreciate you, grieve with you, and celebrate with you. Some call themselves a "very private person" and use that as an excuse for not communicating. When they do not communicate with loved ones, everyone suffers more and those who are left behind grieve more for not having had a chance to grieve along the way and complete their relationship with their loved one while they were still alive and available.

Information that the treatment is not working is available to most patients weeks, even months and occasionally years before their cancer is destined to take their lives, but only if they ask the question bluntly and ask for the unvarnished truth.

Many individuals are not very symptomatic from their cancer at such a point in time. Often, the primary reason they feel bad is the cumulative effects of their treatment when it is not working. Although each treatment may be the same, they are like the blows a boxer receives in a match; by the eighth round each blow takes a greater toll. Just as treatment is intended to have a cumulative beneficial effect against the tumor (if it is working), its toxicities often accumulate (especially when treatment is not working) manifesting themselves in fatigue.

When treatment is working, people recover from treatment toxicity between treatments and will feel better in a stair-step fashion month by month. They may feel a little worse, or at least no better, right after a treatment, but then somewhat better before the next treatment starts. If the stair-steps of your feeling-goods are going down rather than up, your treatment is probably not working and needs to either be changed or stopped. You will feel the stair-steps going down before your doctor can see or measure the trend with scans or blood work, so you have to speak up. An exception to this is when you are on an aggressive treatment, short term (6 month) program aimed at cure where you are hammered over and over and then the treatment ends.

When people stop treatment, most start feeling somewhat, if not dramatically, better for a while, even for weeks or months and occasionally years. If a loss aversion delusion blocks that decision to stop and they decide to continue futile therapy, they can end up losing out on a treatment holiday which could have otherwise been the very best days of the rest of their lives. Futile therapy simply adds its side-effects on top of the cancer symptoms and loads it all on the back of an ever weakening patient. Making a decision not to sacrifice the quality of your life for treatment at such a time turns out not to shorten your life, but in many cases, lengthens it.

> **What you are after is the most symptom-free days. One subtle, often overlooked symptom is time wasted in unnecessary tests and doctor visits.**

I counsel patients that their time is limited and there is nothing they can do to extend whatever that time might be, but they can decide where and how to spend it and how to improve its quality and meaningfulness. Every patient is the master of their fate, the captain of their soul.[15] We know that in most cancer situations, third and fourth line treatment seldom prolongs life, so I invite them to stop it. Many are amazed how much better they feel. Those who stop do so because they have another purpose in their life besides taking treatment and another hope in their life besides just prolonging it. They avoid the loss aversion trap altogether. (See *Windrunners and The Dragon Vanquished*).

Making Important Decisions

- More important than speed in decision making is identifying and focusing on critical pieces of information and goals.
- Focus, focus, focus! Prioritize, prioritize, and prioritize!
- Avoid emotional issues that can preload the brain with emotional heat.
- There is only one way to avoid falling into the loss aversion trap: know about it and watch out for it.

Fighting Through the Near Corner

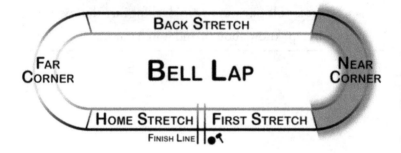

You have had your first treatment and you are going to be taking more until you are in remission or deemed cured and at last get to start down the backstretch. You know what treatment is like and at least that fear which so occupied your thoughts has subsided. Now, you have the time and energy to think about many other things. That can be overwhelming and scary. So let's face them and whittle them down to size.

Chapter 8

Knowing Your Adversaries

The physiologic battle with cancer brings the existential battle with the Dragon, (by whatever names you call it: guilt, fear, anxiety, evil, devil) into the open. The final battle has begun even if the finish line is far off. What is at stake is your heart and without that no one can run a good Bell Lap or endure the physiologic ardors of cancer treatment.

**Cancer is primarily your doctor's responsibility,
but the Dragon is all yours.**

There are some practical things to learn about your physical adversary, cancer, and your psychological/spiritual adversary, the Dragon, which can strike your head with depression and your heart with fear; maybe not yet, but the blows are coming. You have to win the battle in your heart and head so you can best assist the doctor in taking on the battle for your body.

The Big Fear

Running into the near corner it is easy to get tripped up, boxed in or shouldered out by competitors for your attention: the ideas the Dragon throws at you. Its weapon is The Big Fear plus many smaller ones which will nip at your heels. You have been able to manage or outrun them before cancer arrived, but now that you are disconcerted and off balance with a new diagnosis and coming into the near corner of a race you never planned to run, you will find yourself more vulnerable to their tactics.

The Dragon may not confront you head on just yet, but he will offer you escape routes through denial and bargaining. He knows if he can scare you enough maybe you will just drop out of the race altogether, surrender your heart and soul, and shortly thereafter, your life. Depressed people can't take enough treatment to fight off cancer for very long and go down in the record books as DQ (disqualified) or DNF (did not finish)

If you are normal, you will get depressed and it will sap your vitality for a while, but you most likely will not stay that way. Bad news is depressing and only those who are either in denial or crazy don't experience it. Many of us tread through life thinking of our bodies as something we can count on, or we do not think about them at all. We just assume appetite will follow activity, the taste of food will not change, refreshment will follow rest, strength will pretty much endure, biologic functions will be intact, no lumps, no pains, and no panic. But once cancer enters the scene, we no longer know what we can count on and are disconcerted at the very least.

Those who can tolerate their depression and work through it achieve resilience. For them, it is a stimulus to reflect, a way to process their experiences, and thereby gain insight into themselves and life itself. Those who hide from it behind denial become enslaved by it and simply let it grow until the depression destroys them. If it persists and interferes with sleep, work, relationships or treatment, you must ask for help. There are medicines I call stress-busters that can energize you enough to endure it until you can conquer it, and there are counselors who can assist you to navigate the quagmire of feelings that create it.

The Dragon will come up unannounced from behind to overtake you and trip you up. You may need to sprint hard to get away from it, but you have to do it. Take a good look as you pull away because it will bring those feelings back at you over and over in different disguises. The Dragon is a master of deception, but after you have beaten it once, you can see it coming and know how to out run it. Dragons may seem like some fantasy out of children's books, but you are going to meet this one, I guarantee it. The only question is will you recognize it and how you will respond.

Only you can deal with the fear the Dragon will bring. In order to overcome it, you need to recognize every form it takes and every way it impacts your decision making, and hence, your life. This is a bigger deal than most realize. I am not just talking about the big stuff like hurricanes, earthquakes, fires, and terrorism. There are all kinds of fears that seem little, but can ultimately destroy your life.

Fear can do more to shape your life than disease itself. It is the Dragon's mightiest weapon.

One morning I was sharing a cup of coffee with Sue, a wise friend, who had endured arduous treatment for her cancer. She looked great. The clever twinkle had returned to those blue eyes and the effervescence to her smile. Yet, when I asked her how she was doing she replied, "I've been in remission now for two years, and I'm doing better than I expected." Then, with a quick look over her shoulder and almost in a whisper, she added, "But you know, the Dragon is still behind the door! He won't leave me alone and he shows up at the darnedest times."

It was the first time I had heard it put so eloquently, but I had seen it many times before. If you haven't already experienced this, it is likely you will soon know exactly what she's talking about.

So, I want to help you recognize the fears the Dragon will throw at you and how to constructively either avoid or overcome them. You don't need to kill the Dragon and overcome every fear right away, but you must to learn to recognize them and discover what they are doing to you. The Dragon wants to destroy your run and steal your life.

Wherever there is uncertainty the Dragon of fear lurks right behind the door. We scarcely know it is there until relief arrives when it is gone. Little do we recognize its centrality in directing much of our behavior in everyday life before cancer. It doesn't need to rise to the level of tremors, cold sweats, and bounding pulse to steal our joy or manipulate our decisions. The uncertainties of our lives include the insecurity of our jobs, the insufficiency of our bank accounts, the fragility of our relationships, the future of our kids, the strength of our backs, and the keenness of our memory, just to name a few. Then, the diagnosis of a disease beyond our control adds one more huge uncertainty. The cumulative weight squashes many of us and staggers most everyone else.

Our culture applauds the undaunted courage of those who face adversity and never give up, especially if they prevail. Even those who have trembled before it and have moved on in spite of it are heartily acknowledged for their endurance. Fear can be earthshaking whether it is obvious or extremely subtle. It can be blatantly focused on the process of dying, but more often the focus is subconsciously on other things like your unalienable right to life itself and your right to control your life as you see fit.

Rachel told me how pondering the unfairness of it all and all the dreams that would never be, made her furious and got her nowhere. Expressing her feelings helped, but the more she did that the more exhausted and defeated she became. It was only when she let it all go that she could get the Dragon off her back. It wasn't until she accepted the fact that she would never know all the answers to the uncertainties that she could move on with life, make new dreams, and regain the energy and composure she needed to make decisions and take full treatment.

Beware of anger because it can cause you to spin your wheels and go nowhere.

Whether you can identify the source of your fear or not, it can still injure your life or impair your treatment. It is a natural instinctive reflexive response to danger, but in the hands of the Dragon, it can become a bigger deal with deeper roots than it seems at first, so belabor this with me for a while. Go looking for it, and watch your back. The Dragon likes to sneak up on you with it from behind.

We are going to start recognizing the fears the Dragon will throw at you and how to constructively either avoid or overcome them, but first let's address the seduction of denial. If you give into it now, you may ignore everything there is to be said about fear and that will render you clueless and defenseless.

The Great Escape—Denial

When cancer shatters your reality denial offers a seductive escape, but only the truth can pick up the fragments and piece them back together. Finding and accepting your truth is the hardest work of the near corner. Meditate on it, pray about it, and give it full attention. Put all your weight on your left foot of acceptance, and then hurdle denial. Then put your weight on your right foot of hope so you can reach forward to direct the rest of your life and escape the living purgatory that denial creates.

That Dragon is both clever and sinister. Its first tactic is to get you to believe there is nothing to be afraid of (denial). Then it adds false bravado. "I'm smart and the doctors are smart. I'm strong, determined, and courageous. With sheer willpower, I'm going to beat this thing." Denial and bravado are just cover-ups for panic and retreat, glaring signs that the big fear has already got you. Next time you see someone arrogant and brash look for the fear and insecurity beneath; it's there.

Once these defenses have been installed, they create a veneer of safety and security, which in reality is more like putting a Band-Aid over a dirty wound. When the wound disappears from view and you dismiss and deny your prognosis, fear festers producing pus in your life. It starts with the cancer, then spills over and spreads into other areas of your life.

When denial covers over their big fear, many people let their guard down and all kinds of petty fears and insecurities creep in like loss of their status, strength, beauty, athleticism, control, leadership, etc.

Denial doesn't make you immune to fear.
Instead, it is a Band-Aid over it and excuses you
from having to face and deal with it.

Pretending the wolf isn't stalking you does not mean it won't eat you. It only justifies not looking over your shoulder or carrying a gun. How smart is that? I am not saying "accept the bad news, roll over, die, and be happy about it." I am saying that running the bell lap well does not mean giving up the fight or running for your life. It means running towards life rather than away from death. There is a big difference. It starts in your heart which must corral your mind to run, not walk in the right direction. If you lose your heart, your passion and purpose will soon disappear; you may as well be dead already. You can see people like that around every cancer center. They are the Walking Dead (WDs); still moving about but not really living.

Denial says, "There is no bear chasing me."

Everyone's first reaction to bad news is to try to figure out why it is wrong; the tests must be wrong, this is not really happening, or they don't really mean what they said. For cancer, there is no normal length of time for denial to last, but it is clear that the sooner it is overcome the better a bell lap one can run. Let the right foot of hope be the power and the left feet of acceptance provide the balance and agility to get you going in the right direction without falling. Acceptance of the possible bad news is the first step towards meaningful life in spite of it. There are a few different roads to acceptance and a few different ways it can look when you get there. Some are better than others.

Denial is a clever Dragon's weapon and he means to use in one form or another in every segment of the lap to take you out of the running. Just when you think you have beaten it, it can come at you again masquerading in a new disguise, usually of your own creation or occasionally from a "friend." Only critical thinking coupled with the willingness to accept the truth, whatever it might be, will expose how you are fooling yourself. Be ever alert for denial's reappearance and be prepared to walk away again.

Bargaining: Have I got a deal for you!

It may have worked with mom or dad, maybe even with a spouse, but it doesn't work with cancer. None the less, many people improve their behavior just in case an almighty power might reward them with healing grace in exchange. No rabbi, priest or pastor I have spoken with believes that is part of any divine equation, just a dragonish delusion to distract you from reality. Improving behavior is good, just not an effective life-saving strategy to rely on unless it is quitting smoking or meth.

Once you have discarded denial and have left bargaining behind, be ever wary of the fears that recruit denial and bargaining to hide behind. That will get you out of the near corner and into the backstretch.

Draw the Battle Lines

Cancer needs to be fought with every means possible. The illness will affect your life, but don't let it touch your heart. Draw the battle line there. Engage your doctors, question and challenge them, make your decisions, and follow their lead. Don't get your roles confused. Their job is with your body and yours is with your heart. You can make their job more successful by doing yours well. If your heart is safe, then you will be able to cope with the best treatment. Without that, you're toast.

It is normal to feel depressed some of the time when dealing with cancer. It is bad stuff. Only someone in total denial or a crazy person who is out of touch with reality doesn't have such feelings. Normal people sometimes feel like they are losing heart, getting burned out, just too tired to even think, too exhausted to even try, and too discouraged to even consider the possibilities of what I am saying. That is the time to tell your doctor. He can't fight this battle for you, but he can help with medications –the "stressbusters."

These raise the level of natural neurotransmitters in the brain that help us cope with stress and to feel better in spite of it all. They don't eliminate the stress any more than a burst of adrenaline gets rid of the bear that is chasing you. However, the burst of adrenaline helps you outrun the bear. When the bear is cancer, it can keep chasing you day after day, month after month. Adrenaline is short acting and when a burst of it is gone, you need the other long acting neurotransmitters to rise and stay up to enable you to keep running, avoid burnout, sleep well, deal with the illness, and then run some more. Not all of us have enough neurotransmitters to meet the needs that cancer creates. If you are one, get some medicinal help and get back in the battle for your life.

Pharmaceutical companies call these medicines antidepressants because they work well for that, too, but don't let that name disconcert you. Seeing that cancer bear chasing you is depressing. If a little medicine will help you run faster, why not use it? It is not forever. Better running will get you in better shape to cope with all the bear issues now and eventually get you in such good shape you won't need it. Spend some time with a counselor as well. That is not a sign of weakness but of brilliance and determination. The best athletes get sport's counselors, why shouldn't you. Go all in. Why play a game with just one head coach. The best teams have a host of coaches: for the defensive line, the special teams, etc. Etc. Rally your own team of coaches.

Deep Survival

In his book, *Deep Survival*, Gonzalez describes heroes who have survived extraordinary peril. He concludes, "Survival is adaption, and adaption is change, but it is change based upon a true reading of the environment." It is not based on what is hoped for, but what is. It is not based on what is predicted, but what is! Only rapid acceptance of what is makes it possible to conquer any situation whether it's in the cancer center or in the open ocean. So, what follows in the next chapter are common examples of the delusions that sneak into our thinking and can compromise both optimal treatment and a victorious lap. Portraits of acceptance with obstacles that were hurdled are included.

**First, take the time to draw those battle lines
and review these key points:**

- Cancer is primarily your doctor's responsibility, but the Dragon is all yours.

- Fear can do more to shape your life than disease itself. It is the Dragon's mightiest weapon.

- Anger can spin your wheels and cause you to go nowhere.

- Overcoming fear and denial means running towards life rather than away from death.

- Only rapid acceptance of reality makes it possible to conquer any situation whether it's in the cancer center or in the open ocean.

Chapter 9

Lure of the Easy Way

Delusion 1: If I don't accept the truth of my prognosis, I won't have to act accordingly and I'll be fine. (But you can't escape the consequences!)

Delusion 2: If I don't accept the truth of my prognosis, I can escape feeling bad about it. (But it will eat away at your insides!)

Delusion 3: Denying my real prognosis is the only way to be happy. (But just the opposite is true because setting up unrealistic expectations ensures an unhappy crash when they don't pan out and causes anxiety every day until then.)

Delusion 4: If I don't accept the truth of my prognosis, it will be easier for everyone else. (Both true and false. It will be easier for the uncaring and unloving family members and workmates who would rather not deal with your cancer or your feelings. They would prefer a happy, snappy, cheerful albeit deluded you who is carrying on in all your usual functional roles of caring for them and protecting their feelings. But it will be harder for the loving ones who recognize the truth and want to share their genuine feelings, and help you do the same.)

The Eagles described the seduction of the drug culture well, "You can check out any time, but you can never leave."[16] The culture of self-deception is no different.

**You can check out of life with denial any time,
but the truth will never leave!**

Denial's delusion can behave a lot of different ways. It can be defensive, assertive, passive, or passively aggressive. No matter which form it takes, it always crashes. The longer it goes on, the more momentum it builds, the more people around you it recruits, the bigger the crash, and the more people it hurts. The longer it goes on, the more pride gets involved and the harder it is to let it go. It can happen whether there is indeed hope of cure or no rational hope at all. Sometimes, it is overt and other times subtle. Sometimes, it is unconscious and unintentional while other times it is a very conscious and a very intentional defense mechanism. Sometimes, you are dealing with it in yourself and sometimes it is in the people around you.

Kirk was brash acknowledging his chances were slim, maybe only one in 1 million. Then, with an effort at heroism, he would proclaim his intention to be that 1/1,000,000 and would not consider any other possibility, certainly not the more likely 999,000, as if doing so would mark him as a coward or diminish his chances of becoming that exception. He would boast about the existence of outliers with the determination to be one, as if determination was all that was needed. He did not realize this silly charade was trading vitality on the outside for dying on the inside. In doing so, he became ever more disconnected from his reality oriented family and friends. Fear reaped its harvest and the ranks of the WDs added one more and the Dragon won.

It's okay to try hard to be the outlier and we all applaud the courage it takes, but not if it means ignoring the bell lap. You can do both. In my experience, those who run the best bell laps live the longest.

Darlene had missed only one mammogram when she discovered a lump in her left breast. It wasn't that large at 2 cm, but not small. Sadly, under the microscope it's grade was aggressive and scans showed it had already metastasized to her liver. She was talented and much loved, full of zest for life, strong-willed and proud of it. Her energy and assertiveness had brought her many successes and she was determined they would overcome her breast cancer as well. The only way she saw to lead a full life was to deny that the cancer could ever take her life. Hence, she never embraced such thoughts herself or had those conversations with anyone. The subject was unapproachable for everyone at the beginning and so it remained to the end. Sadness and frustration rippled through her family and friends. One lamented, "I was with her often in the final weeks, but I was never able to say good-bye. It just wasn't permitted." What rich and tender conversations were missed! Not only was the door closed to her husband, children, and friends with their expressions of love, but also to their petitions for forgiveness, pleadings for understanding, solace for healing, and offerings for resolution. The disappointed and frustrated left behind often express the greatest sense of loss when a relationship like this has been amputated, incomplete, and unfinished.

It Is Easier, but It Is Not Better

- *It is easier to wallow in self-pity and cash in on the sympathy of kind friends.*
- *It is easier to veer away from facing reality boldly.*
- *It is easier not to think deeply about your life or wrestle with the mysteries of faith.*
- *It is easier to check-out than to check-in to a new upside down life.*
- *It is easier to not even consider the possibility of a new life's purpose in the midst of all the changes.*

- *It is easier to be swept along letting the disease and its treatment control your life than to live meaningfully in spite of it.*
- *It is easier to become attached your cancer and let it become an excuse for every unresolved issue and relationship.*
- *It is easier to let your cancer become a perfect excuse to hide behind or even a weapon to manipulate situations and relationships.*

It is all easier, but it is not better.
Better is harder, but it is better.

Beware the harlots of self-pity, victimhood, and denial who will gladly suck you in with their seductive voices and distract you from honest living. Life with them is never rich and fulfilling. Instead, it is lonely and pitiful because everyone else recognizes what you are doing even if you don't.

The Last Charade

Denial is just as unfortunate when it occurs in your friends and family as it can be in you. In 1629, John Donne wrote, "No man is an island entire of itself; if a clod be washed away by the sea, Europe is less as well as if a promontorie were, as well as if any manner of thy friends or of thine own were; any man's death diminishes me, because I am involved in mankind; and therefore never send to know for whom the Bell tolls; it tolls for thee."[17]

Denial is not your own; it affects us all. Frederick Buechner, expands on those words in, *Listening to Your Life*, "Just as Donne believed that any man's death, when we are confronted by it, reminds us of our common destiny as human beings: to be born, to live, to struggle a while and finally die. We're all in this together."[18]

To deny death is coming is a grand charade and it harms us all. Embracing it will demystify your sense of it in the life cycle and remove a barrier for the rest of us. It won't compel you to run toward it, just temper your need to run away while dragging us along.

Making and pursuing a bucket list can be fun and meaningful to a lot of people if it is not putting a mask on denial. Instead of a celebration of life, it can be just an elaborate way to avoid dealing with the issue. The relief provided by a hedonistic bucket list of extravagant purchases and self-gratifying events is always short lived. When a bucket list intended to make life rich and glorious becomes a distraction from addressing spiritual or relational issues, it will only serve to bankrupt life and expand the corrosive inner turmoil already present.

If you miss the opportunities to invest in the life that awaits you in the backstretch, your life will be the poorer for it, your treatment tolerance less, and your legacy paltry. Research has repeatedly demonstrated that emotional and spiritual health facilitates optimal treatment tolerance and treatment outcome.

Those who accept the Dragon's bucket list delusion, defeat themselves. Make your bucket list a meaningful celebration that enriches relationships and it will endure in the hearts of many.

Kick the Bucket List if it is a gift from a Dragon.

Ignorance Is Not Bliss

Aware that everyone is watching, some patients who are too proud to get real, quietly step over their cancer like a crack in the sidewalk and keep on moving into life as if nothing has happened. They have no idea how to act, so they begin an ever more elaborate charade of nonchalance. Their carefree all-is-under-control act on the outside is masking the growing torment on the inside. This is particularly true of those who look for their identity in the eyes of others. Those who choose such intentional blindness have a surprise crash landing waiting for them. If you lack the emotional vocabulary and confidence to process what you are feeling, you may stagger off in one phony direction after another. You need a counselor and soon, or it will be too late for a meaningful bell lap.

A counselor is a luxury you deserve at this time in your life.

Some disguise their fear by casting their denial in the high and heroic terms of protecting others. Denial is never heroic and casting it as protection of others is a sham. Our children and contemporaries need compassionate reality as soon as possible to give them time to process, grieve, and celebrate. It also gives them a chance to mature, lend support, and to complete or resolve their relationships. Without it, confusion reigns and distance grows between loved ones. It is sad to watch. Those in denial think they're fooling everyone, but everyone else sees right through their bedraggled and pathetic performance. Fear beats the drum, and they dance, but nobody enjoys watching it.

Sometimes, everyone in the family gets involved in denial trying to protect each other and in the process everyone is silenced. The elephant in their hearts may be pleading for true emotional interaction, but has no voice. When it is a long-standing family pattern for dealing with illness, it needs to be deconstructed and replaced. Anyone who can climb over the wall of denial can coach the rest. If you do, you can change the future and the lives of your children's children will benefit.

Throw Yourself in the Dark Hole

Thoughts about what you are losing are unavoidable (and normal), but denial is no escape. Grief will always have its way with you. It will come out one way or another, often at most inconvenient times. It is a spoiler, and unless you deal with it, every day will be in peril, like driving on bald tires—spin out can be around any corner. Get help. What you still have is too valuable to waste. Dredge up every feeling from that dark hole where they hide, bring them into the light, discover them completely, embrace them, and deal with them.

Amyotrophic Lateral Sclerosis (ALS) doesn't take a life suddenly; it steals it little by little, one day at a time, until there's nothing left. It gives you plenty of time to reflect as you watch strength seep away and death approach. This was Prof. Morrie Schwartz's experience,[19] and he left some good advice. "By throwing yourself into these emotions, by allowing yourself to dive in, all the way, over your head even, you experience them fully and completely. You know what pain is. You know what love is. You know what grief is."

You know what loss is. You discover what you will miss and what you will regret. Think about it all. Talk about it. Write about it. Be angry about it. Then deal with it, on your knees, on the counselor's couch, or over a cup of coffee with a dear friend. Then put it away until next time and walk boldly into the life you still have.

When you discover what grief is, you can discover what it is not and that is even more important. It isn't you! You still have you. Enjoy what you have. Keep the illness/Dragon in its place and move on. Suffering and loss deserve their do, but no more than that. They are what they are, but they do not preclude meaningful, productive, and even joyful living. Put them in their place again and again and keep moving onward.

This is not something you can, or should, do by yourself. You need another—a spouse, a sibling, a friend, a pastor, or a counselor. Odds are that someone is already at your side and experiencing your illness with you. If not, find someone. People in isolation move forward slowly or not at all. Conversation can heal all parties. The dark and potholed roads you are traveling will come to everyone someday, so they will be better off for having navigated them with you.

Every hope and fear, every attempt to make sense of your illness, every revelation, and every roadblock deserves attention. What you discover will define the challenges of the backstretch that is before you. Many obstacles will yield answers to questions. Much of the turmoil will be resolved. What you feared will lose its power and your need for denial will lessen.

A Buddhist I knew would say about life's issues, "Identify them, and then detach from them. Pretend as if they don't exist." As I watched him do that, what first appeared to be serenity soon revealed itself as a cold lifelessness with a benevolent, but artificial smile. The passion and tenderness to relate to others, and the eagerness to find meaning and purpose were all gone. While waiting to die, he didn't need denial because he seemed in many ways to be dead already.

Detachment looked different on the outside from denial, but the effect was the same–loneliness!

We will explore some action strategies in the next chapter, but first get rid of those delusions once and for all!

- You can check out with denial any time, but the truth will never leave!
- Beware the harlots of self-pity, victimhood, and denial who will gladly suck you in with their seductive voices and distract you from honest living.
- To deny death is coming is a grand charade and it harms us all. Embracing it will demystify your sense of it in the life cycle and remove a barrier for the rest of us.
- Kick the Bucket List if it is a gift from the Dragon.
- A counselor is a luxury you deserve at this time in your life.

Chapter 10

Action Strategy

Letting Go and Grabbing On

"Last night I had a nightmare," a mother of three in tennis shoes and a gym outfit told me "I don't remember all of it. I just remember walking around in a daze and falling over a cliff only to catch hold of a branch in mid fall. Hanging on for dear life I was wrestling with different voices in my head: some saying hang on and others pleading, 'Just let go.' I woke up still fighting with that question and realized it was all about my cancer. Should I fight or should I give up?"

This was a forty-five-year-old woman whose lymphoma had just relapsed. Her original treatment had been very difficult and she was just rising out of the fog of her last chemo with so much of her life yet unfinished before her. Now, she was facing relapse with the specter of even more treatment or probably death not too far away.

It struck me that her nightmare capsulated just how many cancer patients see their conundrum. Either fight or give up. Either spit in the face of death one more time or accept it. Hang on or let go. However, it need not really be an either/or situation. You can hang on with one hand and let go with the other. Not many people can do that unless they know what else to grab onto before they let go. I told her to do both.

Fight with everything you've got for your life, but give up on your need to have it. Escape from the threat of the fear wielding Dragon and walk free.

Needers and Wanters

There's nothing wrong with *wanting* more life, but *needing* it is something quite different. It is the difference between being a free human being and being an addict. The *Wanters* saver a slice of life every day without the fear that it will be their last, whereas the *Needers* are so busy fearing there won't be enough days left to even enjoy what days they still have. *"Not Enough" is the welcome sign* that invites the Dragon in and gives it the power to consume their thoughts with angst and manipulate their behavior.

Not even a good treatment plan is enough for the *Needers;* the Dragon is always there. They may not be able to see him, but they can always feel him. Those who are in touch with their feelings tell me, "He is so real you can almost smell him." However, when they give up *needing* their life, everything changes. The Dragon loses its power over them and they get more of the real thing every day—delicious life without fear. Sounds like mumbo-jumbo! Such a paradox, but it is true. Just ask the ones who have experienced it. The real question is how did they do it? Read on, they will tell you.

Most of us have been in control of our decisions most of the time. When you make the *letting go of life* decision you gain control of something else: your thoughts. The one who is addicted to this life is nearly powerless to control his thoughts. He must always be on guard to protect himself from fear and anxiety. Will the treatment work? How long will it work? Will it interfere with my life or my appearance, what will people think? As soon as he lets his guard down, wham, a discouraging, life-threatening thought floods in, "What if, what if, and what if?"

Odds are you have had such thoughts yourself at all kinds of unexpected moments and especially in the middle of night. The fear of losing control of some aspect of your life can be a 24-hour proposition. Denial requires a continuous and conscious effort to negate facts and feelings. It is a lot of work, requiring a lot of energy. It is a somewhat effective defense during the waking hours, but it doesn't work at night. Any incongruity between the real facts and our constructed beliefs will destroy our rest at night and dampen the joy of play in our days.

I have had people tell me, "Sure that makes sense but it is pretty ridiculous. I can't do that. It would mean giving up hope. I've got to have hope." Yes, hope is essential, but the letting go I am speaking of does not abandon hope. Instead, it expands it. The abandoning only happens if you choose detachment or resignation by letting go without something to grab on to. Instead of just giving up and dangling there staring into the abyss, you can let go of the control you never had and grab onto something else, something better. That is what the Windrunners do. (See *Bell Lap Windrunners and the Dragon Vanquished*.)

Identify It So You Can Defeat It

Cancer actually can help in the universal human plight of dealing with fear by bringing it out in the open where it can be confronted and dealt with, but some stealthy fears will still try to remain hidden. Most people have to drill down to see where fears have invaded the different arenas of their lives. Many people have been protected by a veneer of the good life, status, possessions or health such that they have been able to overlook the taunting of the Dragon or compensate for the wounds it inflicts. Fear is only something they read about or see in others; it is not real to them. Yet, it can still be there manipulating their thoughts, decisions, and actions. It just moves unrecognized in their lives beneath the veneer.

Identify your big fears, and write them down. Make a list and give each fear a name. Then go in search of every other little fear, even the ones that are so small that you hesitate to call them fear at all. Write them down, too. Go looking in every part of your life and don't let any fear hide behind any euphemism like *concerned about* or *troubled by* or *maybe*.

Then start imagining about how each one can hurt you and how they can collectively box you in and start eroding your life. Think long and hard about how they influence your decisions, your expectations, and your happiness. Ask yourself how you would feel and what you might do if you weren't afraid of them. Write the answers down and mull them over. Drag the Dragon into the open and expose every tooth and claw. Then you are at least able to keep an eye on him and out run him whenever he tries to overtake you. If you see him coming, you can out pace him and hold him off until you can defeat him later.

Find your fear, name it, and keep your eye on it. After watching it for a while and seeing what it is doing to your life, get ticked off enough to do something about it. Learn some tricks of how to manage fear and buy yourself enough time to figure out how to altogether defeat it. Those who are able to get fear off their backs lighten their load, run faster, better, and often longer down the backstretch, and even enjoy the running.

Being good will not get the Dragon to leave you alone; there is nothing in it for him. However, indifference, especially mocking indifference is something he cannot abide. Your task will be to figure out what you need to do to be able to ignore him. You do that and he becomes irrelevant, powerless, defeated, and will recede into the darkness from whence he came. The Windrunners do it and you can, too. Remember: It's not denying he is out there, it's not denying a disease threatens your life, it's not giving up caring. It's having a game plan he can't spoil.

It caught my attention and piqued my curiosity when I didn't see fear in some of my patients. They would walk and not be faint. They would run and not grow weary. They would smile and I didn't know why. I couldn't tell whether something called them forward, or something lifted them from behind. I came to think of them as the Windrunners because they ran faster, smoother, and longer, as if lifted over the rocks and potholes on the track of their cancer journey. I started watching for what was different about them.

It is essential that you figure out what you are up against, what your own personal war on terror looks like, and where it comes from. It's not the biological war taking place in the cancer center, but the one in your heart, in the shadows, in the dark, quiet, all-alone-times between your thoughts. It seemed the Windrunners had done that.

Beware of Arrogance

I once went to a shrink to help me cope with a problem of loss. Counseling was a fascinating experience and I learned a lot. Somewhere during that time, the psychiatrist said to me, "You are anxious." My response was, "No way! You're wrong. Not me. You are way off base there." I think his unspoken reaction was probably, "Whoa, another blind bozo masquerading as a know-it-all." Then he said patiently, "Okay, but why don't you try this pill and see if you feel a lot better, trust me on this." I was thinking, "Alright. I'll humor him, but I'm not anxious. I am successful and I am at the top of my game. People come to me for advice. Besides, I've seen what anxiety looks like in other people and that's not me." I was also probably thinking, "It's not cool to be anxious, definitely not manly, not going there."

Well, I took the pill and pretty soon I felt, slept, and functioned a whole lot better. It was great. The anxiety that I thought I didn't have was gone. I readily confessed, "Okay, Doc, you're right and you have my attention. Now let's figure out why I'm so anxious, and what I'm afraid of. I want to get rid of it so I can get off that pill and on with life." So, I learned what fear looks like to me. When I did, I started seeing it in my patients masquerading as all kinds of less embarrassing totally phony things. I encourage you not to be as arrogant as I was and assume this topic only applies to other people.

Fear is probably playing a lot bigger role in your life than you imagine. It does for most everyone, admittedly in some more than others. I caution you against assuming you are the one with less fear until you have really taken a good look because it is you who has something to gain. Most people fear death and a host of other things. So, trust me and humor me a bit while we talk about those fears other people have and see, if perchance, any of them are yours as well.

Confidence in your known and proven strengths won't help you much when you face an enemy that has been around for a long time, like fear. Fear's first tactic is to convince you that there's nothing to be afraid of. Its second tactic is to convince you that you're not really afraid.

While most of us would shun another's duplicitous word or action, often that is exactly how we behave ourselves. We pretend to think and feel one way while behaving another. The disconnect is between our words, which sound so good, and our behavior that belies them. Pride lets us live in the apparent bravado of our words rather than dealing with the quagmire of our feelings. When words mask the fears inside, the fears simply reign unchecked to haunt, manipulate, steal our joy, and cripple our run. It is easier to recognize and confess the fears in our hearts if we know there is a solution and a way to overcome them. There must be, because the Windrunners have done it.

Getting Real with Yourself Comes First

An especially valid fear which we seldom recognize is of a disassembling, a coming apart of all the façades that we have created to give us self-worth. Deep down we are afraid that we will be found out for who we really are. Disease or misfortune can do that. Often we don't really know who we are, but we are afraid that we aren't good enough. If we are much loved, those awful feelings are less acute but not gone. Since mid-adolescence, most of us have been developing a whole repertoire designed to win approval in our families, among our peers at work, in the community, at church, and at play. It is hard enough to orchestrate all these roles when we are healthy and life is going smoothly, but it really gets challenging when illness or disability sets in. While intellect often remains, energy often declines. Then passion, fitness, and creativity leave making the cover-up act more difficult. The solution is to get real now so you don't have to do it later when you can't. Surrounding yourself with the people who enjoy and value the real you is a good place to start. Just let the others, the posers, go and you will have one less thing like keeping up an act, to be afraid of later.

George was a fiercely independent man in his mid-sixties. He had a swarthy face, with chiseled features and a lean muscular frame, regularly toned by his demanding physical work. Around his family he was aloof, arrogant, and controlling. Their responses to him were respectful and compulsory. Unfortunately, his smoking had caught up with him and landed him in a skimpy bun-revealing gown in a hospital bed with lung cancer. The mass on his x-ray was small and operable with a reasonable chance of cure. However, George hated hospitals and detested the indignity and loss of control that cancer had thrust upon him. He chose to continue his control charade that everyone seemed to buy into and to go home to die rather than submit to an operation and the humiliation of a dependent hospital stay. He became evermore taciturn and withdrawn, ever playing the role of macho man, somehow heroic in his own eyes, right to the end. He was a very lonely terrified man hiding in his bravado.

If one's dignity depends on the façades of an artificial self, then the odds are it will be uncovered and lost. If self-worth depends upon what you can physically accomplish, that will be lost, too. If beauty is all about what others see of you on the outside, then your Cinderella clock is approaching midnight. It is time to get real and find friends who value authenticity and then give it to them. They are the ones you want to be with you in the foxhole.

Mildred never did. She was an attractive, but lonely woman in her early seventies. I suspect she'd always been naturally attractive, but it was hard to say as she was so prim, prepped, painted, and coiffed whenever I saw her. Clearly, she spent a great deal of time and got a lot of attentive help before ever going out in public. She insisted on appointments after 1 P.M. to allow enough time for cosmetics. What she achieved was tasteful and stylish, but her beauty didn't radiate. There was nothing inside that glowed. I'm sure there is a story beneath, but it was well concealed.

Except for her breast cancer, she was remarkably healthy. She was financially solvent and blessed with capable grown children and grandchildren who were never around. Little wonder, as her focus was entirely on herself and keeping up appearances. She could find nothing else to live for. We could see her cancer on x-rays, but her only symptoms were those of aging. However, her cancer became her excuse for checking out of life, and she did. It was not the cancer that started in her breast that took her, but a cancer of fear and insecurity that had long ago started in her soul. She just seemed to evaporate.

Take Control and End it All

One alternative is, of course, Physician-Assisted Suicide or a poison recipe off the internet. The proponents of such champion the sense of control it gives and the preservation of dignity it ensures. They champion the avoidance of writhing in pain, losing bodily functions, messing with bleeding wounds or babbling in delirium. My thirty years of hospice experience attests that those things seldom ever happen and never with so much theater. Every Hemlock Society* orchestrated death confirms the deadly power of fear. (*A society committed to orchestrating death has adopted the name of the poisonous Hemlock tea drank by Socrates 399BC.)

Alice had lung cancer. It was metastatic and of the sort that usually takes people's lives quickly. However, when I met her she had already had it for two years without the cancer growing much or causing any symptoms. Her weight was stable, appetite intact, and her usual smokers cough remained unchanged for years. There were no clinical signs of cancer. Curiously, she had been a Hemlock member for many years dating back to when she was a young mother. She had accumulated all the necessary ingredients to end her life and had carefully hidden them away for that fateful day, so that she could orchestrate her final exit.

One might think that such careful preparation would produce comfort and peace, even a sense of empowerment in knowing the ultimate control of life was securely in her own hands, but it didn't. It didn't create the carefree spirit she sought. Instead, this miserable woman, whom I cared for over a course of years, was anything but free. She was so ravaged by fear that she became obsessed with the details of taking her life. Instead of reveling in freedom from symptoms and the stability of her non-progressive disease, she worried about making a mistake while killing herself. What if it didn't work? What if it left her alive, but disabled? The day before she killed herself, I examined her and found no evidence of her cancer, but found every evidence of her riveting fear. She was riddled with it and had transmitted it to her only her son, both were truly among the walking dead. A life that could have been meaningful for months, perhaps years, was sabotaged by fear. Control is not the answer; it's a mirage.

Not all fears are so dramatic but all are destructive. Whatever flavors you have sampled so far, you're destined to meet a veritable smorgasbord of new ones dealing with cancer. Some will come from symptoms, some from doctors, some from the tests, others from the media, and still others from unwitting friends. It doesn't matter where fear comes from, whether it is out of your past or in your present. It doesn't matter if it's imaginary or exaggerated. It's all real when you experience it and must be discovered and dealt with or you will die with it and very possibly transmit it to your kids.

It is one of the most primordial driving forces of our human existence which normally acts as a natural safety and alarm mechanism, but must be modulated by reason. However, reason is limited by knowledge and knowledge is limited by experience. As children, we had parents for protectors until we accrued enough knowledge and experience. Of course, that only worked as long as we trusted them enough to listen. Once grown and out on our own, some suggest that God reserves that role for Himself, but is equally limited by whether we trust Him enough to listen.

What's It Feel Like?

When fear overrules reason, it poisons your intellect.

The Dragon can just use fear to mess with you or to really take you out. Studies have shown that 90 percent of people put under severe stress are not able to think clearly or solve simple problems. Creativity, insight, cool thinking, and the rational reflection that are necessary for a measured response to a problem are severely impaired by fear.

When fear poisons your spirit, the physiologic response can be the same as when bacteria poisons your bloodstream: sweating, racing pulse, dry mouth, dizziness, and even delirium. Your head gets a message that something is terribly wrong. You can almost smell it, then comes a strange brassy taste on the tongue, and agitated feelings of *need to do something, but I don't know what, need to run but don't know where.*

Broadcaster, Tony Snow, while wrestling with colon cancer, cautioned, "We need to get past anxiety. The mere thought of dying can send adrenaline flooding through our system. A dizzy, unfocused panic seizes you. Your heart pumps; your head swims. You think of nothing and swoon. You fear partings; you worry about the impact on family and friends. You fidget and get nowhere."

Fear, whatever flavor, is a big deal all on its own. You have to nail this one. Treatment of the cancer depends upon you controlling your fear. Running the bell lap well depends upon you defeating it.

Keeping Fear in the Open

Acute fears can be medicated so you will feel better and think better, but they don't go away. You still have to deal with them or they just go underground and become chronic which is when they are the most destructive. They can lie dormant like the seeds of knapweed tracked into the mountain meadow on hikers' boots. Those seeds wait for the warm rains of spring to germinate like dormant fears lie in wait for the next sign of relapse. At the opportune moment, the seeds and the fears both burst forth into full bloom. The unseen roots of the knapweed give off a toxin that prevents healthy plants from germinating nearby and whole meadows are taken over and destroyed. When dormant fear germinates in anyone, it can poison meaningful living, destroy dreams, squelch passions, spoil relationships, interfere with sleep, and sap energy. All in all, they just drain the joy out of life. Don't let your fears go underground. Find them, confront them, talk about them openly, and get help dealing with them.

David understood the universal impact of the fear of death when he penned the 23rd Psalm, "Yea though I walk through the valley of the shadow of death." His choice of metaphor is powerful and accurate. Death casts a long shadow. David didn't say the doorway of the shadow or the shadow of the pillar of death. He said the valley of the shadow of death. A valley is cast into shadow by a mountain. The mountain is fear.

While death from cancer takes but an instant, its shadow extends back months and years. Walking that valley takes a long, often lonely time. Even friends and family at one's side can't change the fact that dying is a singular business. Yet, through the years I have noticed there are some who seemed to be neither afraid nor alone which sparked my curiosity. Again it was the Windrunners.

Prison Walls

We look around at those who have disabling phobias like the fear of heights or tight places or spiders and we think it is strange. The agoraphobic confines himself at home for fear of going outside. His world shrinks and avoidance behaviors reign. The fear of death does the same thing and imprisons many with walls that are hard to see. Both new and old relationships are walled off because they are perceived as too painful, and what's the point? New endeavors are walled off because there might not be time to finish. Travel and adventure are walled off because one might get sick or die along the way. Asking for help or special consideration at work and home can be walled off out of fear of being rejected or becoming a burden. Going out in public or social events can be walled off by vanity or the fear of embarrassing side effects. None of these walls need exist, yet I have known patients who lived small lives behind these poisonous walls. Sometimes, they were walls inherited from their parents, sometimes built by friends, or by dramatizations in the media.

It's the What-Ifs that build the walls.

They are the imagination's questions that are always knocking at the door of tomorrow's unknowns. They are the breath of the Dragon whispering nightmares in the dark—even to those in remission. Sometimes, they are things the doctor said or didn't say which could have been clarified on the spot but weren't. Some are a riptide of confusing lab reports or new symptoms that whipsaw your helpless emotions. Sometimes, they are the contagion of your neighbor's fear casually offered, *"What if?"* When you collect enough of them, you can build your own prison and crawl inside.

Curiously, some people hear the same whispers, but remain immune. They experience the limitations from their cancer, but not from fear. They seem to know something that the rest of us don't.

For the some, the legion of death's fears vanquishes all efforts to retain control and invites resignation, despair, and cynicism.

They die quietly and uneventfully at home or in a hospital. None are in control, all succumbing to that which cannot be avoided any longer, most having accepted their fate and are just too tired to be terrified any longer, numb from being uncertain for so long.

Some observers kid themselves in describing a numb death as peaceful, when in reality it is just plain exhaustion. The difference is readily apparent to anyone who has seen both. A numb death is nothing like a peaceful one. I've been watching for years. The difference seems to have to do with bliss, surrender, and trust.

Those who die in peace seemed to have something spiritual going on that doesn't require their control or understanding. It is something that apparently transcends human knowledge, yet is humanly knowable and redefines for them what others call "the end." Perhaps, it is that same thing that brought purpose and energy to their whole bell laps, revealed one step at a time right up to the end. Even hospital staff just passing through their room to check vital signs or draw blood would come out saying, "There's something special going on with the patient in room 302."

Fight with everything you've got for your life, but give up on your need to have it. Escape from the threat of the fear wielding Dragon and walk free by taking the time to do these few things.

- Identify your big fears, write them down, and give each fear a name.

- Then go in search of every other little fear, even the ones that are so small that you hesitate to call them fear all. Write them down, too.

- Go looking in every part of your life and don't let any fear hide behind any euphemism like concerned about or troubled by or maybe.

- Then start imagining about how each one can hurt you and how they can collectively box you in and start eroding your life.

- Think long and hard about how they influence your decisions, your expectations, and your happiness.

- Ask yourself how you would feel and what you might do if you weren't afraid of them.

- Write the answers down and mull them over.

Chapter 11

Combat Fear Action Plan

Begin a Counter Insurgency

I t starts with defense. You have got to protect yourself before you can go on the offensive. Start by focusing. Navy Seal, Mike Owen, recalled, "The only way I could endure the hardship and control my anxiety through seal training was by focusing on just making it to the next meal."[20] This is pretty good advice for us as enduring cancer treatment is just about as close as we will get to seal training.

Focus only on what is knowable and necessary for today. Don't sacrifice today to what is uncertain in the future.

Dave had high-grade prostate cancer and was on aggressive treatment. His sweetheart and wife, Lisa, had every reason to be afraid of what might happen to him. She told me, "I discovered when I focused only on today, I could do alright, just as scripture says to do!" She described that when she disciplined herself to focus only on today's decisions, using only today's information, that there wasn't room for anxious thoughts about the uncertainties of tomorrow to creep in. She emphasized how much discipline it took to achieve this, to just refuse to think about whether Dave would be around to attend their children's weddings or meet the grandkids, ride out into the mountains, or any number of future plans and dreams. The more she threw her energy and her thoughts into what she was going to do that very day, the better she did. It was a self-taught lesson that she had to learn over and over again.

Deciding on a plan and taking action to implement it decreases fear.

Make plans for your week and your day, but each morning focus on what you want to do in the next hour or before your next nap. Assess your energy, make a plan, and then do it. You can always alter your plans as new information becomes available. Sometimes, the plan is to get a second opinion or take time to research, ponder, pray, take a trip or start a project. Whatever it is, explicitly identify it, write it down, give it a timeframe, and start working on it. That makes it real. Then update it. Just knowing you have a plan, even a short term plan to just gather more information, will keep fear at bay. Looking back at the plans you made and followed will give you confidence that you can keep doing it.

Getting lost alone in the mountains in the dark has been a fear laboratory for me. I'm afraid of the dark and I don't like being alone, but it invariably happens every year when I am out bow hunting for elk. I feel like a six-year-old scared of bears and wolves and cougars and whatever else might be out there in the dark—all those things people rarely ever see. I have discovered how reassuring it is to find a trail that is going in the right direction. It is usually a game trail which peters out after a while, but with a headlamp, one can see a bit of the trail. Just seeing some trail and having a short term plan really helps. It is the same with cancer. Make your short term plan

Beware: Fear Is Contagious

> **Avoid fearful people. Don't give them any airtime; none at all.**

Surround yourself with safe people. Be on the lookout for the dangerous ones that are often uncomfortable talking about life with cancer. They will default to expressing their sympathy or their fears, or to telling you about someone else who died or had a terrible experience. It is exceedingly unlikely that someone else's cancer experience will biologically match your own even if it is the same type. It is more likely that their story will be a source of confusion or alarm. Unless your friend brings an encouraging story about someone's inspiring, triumphant life in spite of cancer, change the subject. All their other stories are just anxiety-fodder for the Dragon to feed you. You don't need it.

Be prepared, interrupt them, and change the subject. Ask them a question about themselves or tell them about some other aspect of your life. Be intentional in initiating conversation about the rest of your life. It will help sustain your relationships. Many people are uncomfortable talking about cancer and run out of things to say pretty fast, so you need to be prepared to redirect them. Understand that their discomfort comes from fear and ignorance. If you are afraid, they will be, too. If you are relaxed, they will usually follow your lead. You can take control and help them be comfortable around you. Otherwise, you can experience a growing sense of loneliness and disengagement from life if such people avoid you to protect their own relational inadequacies. Save both of you and your relationship by steering conversation into other topics.

Beware of the Internet

There is more on the Internet to confuse, mislead, and alarm you then to help you. The problem is not the absence of information, but your inability to glean and understand precisely what is pertinent to your specific type, subtype, stage, and grade of your cancer, and to separate it from irrelevant and misleading stuff. You've already hired an expert who spent years gathering just the information you're looking for and ferreting out what precisely applies to your unique situation. Use him/her. Be demanding about what you need to know.

More often than not I've seen patients more confused and more scared after their searches on the Internet that took them rambling to all kinds of inapplicable and confounding data. If you are going to go there, you must know the details of your cancer. Resist reading about anything that doesn't exactly correspond to your precise situation. One patient told me, "The more I learn the more questions I have and I am unable to evaluate it all. The more I read the more fear I have."

While I am a strong encourager of self-advocacy and taking personal responsibility for one's health, my best advice for the fearful is to find a good doctor. Ask him the tough questions. Let him/her give you the answers that are tailored to your individual situation. Cancers of the same type can behave dramatically differently in different people. Consequently, only someone who knows the unique biology that is in you can tell you what to expect. If your doctor doesn't have the time and skill to answer your questions, he probably won't take the time or have the skill to treat it well either. So, move on and find another. Then let the expert physician be the doctor. You focus on being the patient and taking on the illness and the Dragon.

Fake It

Theodore Roosevelt wrote in his diary during his trips into the wilderness, "There were all kinds of things of which I was afraid, but by acting as if I was not afraid, I gradually ceased to be afraid." This is effective, but it takes forcefully averting one's mind from frightening thoughts. It works provided you know it is only an act for temporary survival and not a disguise for denial.

William Wallace, the Scotsman with the blue painted face immortalized by Mel Gibson in the movie, Braveheart, rallied his thirteenth century Scottish Highlanders against the tyrannical English by reminding them that, "a life lived in fear is no life at all." We all will die one day, but to succumb to fear is to give up your freedom and without that you may as well be dead already. Cancer uses fear to steal your freedom and your life long before it takes your body. Muster courage, and when you can't, fake it. That is a good strategy to have in your repertoire, at least in a pinch. Realize, though, that it is only for the short term. There is a better long term strategy.

Distract Your Mind

My niece, Julie, taught us all something about how to deal with fear last summer when we were climbing Mt. Rainier again. Family tradition dictates that when the kids reach sixteen, they can join the family rope team up the glaciers. She was a cute, vivacious kid with braces and huge brown eyes, a stark contrast to the strapping brutes that preceded her. Sons, nephews, and dads all rallied to give Julie a shot at the summit. She was harnessed up and roped to climb through the one AM darkness on a precipitous route that serpentines around crevasses, below grand seracs (huge blocks of ice), and over ice bridges on the mountain's southern flank. A tumult of questions vented her anxiety as we climbed, but never compromised the "can-do attitude" that propelled her and helped hold fear at bay.

After summiting at dawn and returning to our tents lower on the Ingram glacier, her feelings came tumbling out, "Unc, I was scared the whole time! I always felt as if I was about to fall. Fear of the unknown in the dark is the worst!"

When I asked her how she managed, she responded, "I decided to think about something else. I tried different things. I thought about them in great detail like I was writing an editorial.

Thinking about other things didn't really interfere with what I had to do like keep my crampons flat on the ice, feet apart, and step, step, step. However, those other thoughts left no room for the terror to settle in."

Wow! I had to write that down. She wasn't in control over her circumstances, but she took control of her thoughts! I had stumbled onto the same thing when I was face-to-face with a grizzly bear in the Yukon. I know it works at least for the short term.

Find a Partner in Fear and Declaw It!

One hundred years ago and 8,000 miles away, a fatherless twelve-year-old, Françoise, was discovering the lessons of life by observing the raw realities of existence as it played out in the bush country of South Africa. His much admired Uncle Mopani was his mentor. As they traveled the Okavango Delta, the land of the lion, cheetah, and elephant, the darkness deepened and the bird songs seemed to become frenzied with desperation and foreboding. Francoise whispered softly to Mopani about his fear as if the very words would make it worse. Mopani replied, "I'm a bit frightened myself." This admission from one of the bravest men Françoise had ever met calmed his own fear and raised Mopani immeasurably in his estimation

---

**Nothing feeds fear as much as the pretense
that it has no valid cause to exist.**

Mopani's admission of fear not only confirmed the validity of Françoise's, but also, "by abolishing all pretense between them, made them partners in fear, removing the greatest dread of all; that one would be left to deal with fear on one's own."[21]

You have to exercise some discretion in choosing with whom you will share your fear to avoid just creating a fear fest. Sometimes, an objective friend is best rather than a spouse in order to avoid potentiating their own fears. Other times a spouse is perfect. Share it all, even the fear that invades your sleep or back slaps you in the midst of the day. Somehow, sharing lessens the sting.

Lisa described how she needed a "full disclosure agreement" with Dave about his cancer and her fears. She just wanted him to know and needed the freedom to tell him, but she discovered something more. When she voiced her fears, she tamed them and they lost their power!

Techniques for Fear Management

Naming the Dragon saps its power, like singling out an enemy and facing them head on—"I see you, I know you, and

I'm going to take you on." Fear doesn't like too much attention. When it is free to wander the back roads of your consciousness day and night, it is the happiest and does the most harm. But identified, spoken of, confronted, and shared, it shrinks in size and you can apply your weapons of reason, humor, distraction, and prayer to it.

I vividly recall getting manual physical therapy on my stiff and painful neck from old football injuries. The therapist fingers would try to wrench my frozen vertebrae into motion. In so doing, he caused me the most excruciating pain I had ever experienced. I guess I was kind of a wimp about pain, like a lot of men who have never given birth. Watching the beads of sweat forming across my forehead, my grimace, and white knuckles, John cavalierly said, "It's just pain, Rob. It's not forever and it's not killing you. Get over it!" That was obvious, I suppose, but I laughed and somehow it was different after that. He said it to be funny, but there was as much truth in it as there was humor.

The same applies to fear. It's just fear. It's not killing you. Get on with your life and laugh at yourself whenever you can. It will help. You need lots of little techniques like this to deal with fear because you never know when or where is going to pop up. That's normal. You are not defective or cowardly when it does.

Sometimes the Dragon is more like an octopus. I used to wrestle them in college to eat and to sell. The trick was to hold one's breath, glide in quietly, unseen, and tackle the octopus before it could get its arms attached to the rocks on the bottom. Invariably, it would get some tentacles attached to something and I was left trying to pull off one arm after another. Every time I pulled up one and turned to the next, the first would reattach— often to me or my mask or my air hose. Fear is like that. You no sooner deal with it in one arena than it attacks you in another. The different techniques are useful and can help you cope, but what you really need to do is take out that whole octopus, all the fears, the whole Dragon. Not even completing treatment and being declared disease-free will do that. The Windrunners did it, some even before the treatment started.

Taking treatment for cancer is also a lot like fighting a lion. Traveling in Kenya, I met a Maasai warrior, a game guide who had dramatic scars all over his arms, neck, chest, and back. In vivid detail, he described how a lion had attacked one of his cattle. When he thrust a spear in its side, the lion had turned on him. A wrestle to the death ensued leaving him the victor, but critically wounded. The lion was dead, her throat slit by his machete. When I asked how he felt during the encounter, he replied that the situation left no room for fear, only for the determination to meet the task at hand. However, fear moved in with incapacitating trembling of body and spirit once the lion was dead.

As I heard his story, it reminded me of many patients some cured by surgery alone and others who, having endured the onslaught of their cancer and treatment, described how an almost disabling fear had moved in when it was all over. One said as long as she was focused on the fight, there was no time for fear, but that once the fight was over, "Fear was having its way with me. I could think of nothing else, but what I had been through and what I might have to face again." The Dragon was behind every door! At work, at home, on vacation, during the day, and at night.

The mind, once cleared of its all-absorbing battle focus, is a fertile field for growing something else. Before seedlings of fear can take root, it is important to plant new ideas and new intentions to give the mind something to nurture and grow.

Fear loves a vacant mind and quickly moves in uninvited. Don't let the relief of completing treatment leave your thoughts empty. Fill them with something meaningful that leaves no room for fear. Not just new activities but new ideas. That is a critical element of the backstretch.

Jim, a marathon runner and young father with testicular cancer, proudly told me, "I've been in remission now for two years and just now am becoming less fearful." By this, he meant that his life had filled up again with enough normal things and his medical appointments were sufficiently far apart that he wasn't constantly reminded of his disease.

Then he confessed he used to dread looking in the mirror or washing his body. Any new spot or thickening of the skin, any new ache or hint of a lump would trigger panic. In other words, fear was still alive and in total control, just not always in view; the Dragon had gone underground. Then something changed.

"Fear is not something you negotiate with or try to control or ignore," he said. "It's a bully. It won't go away until you stare it in the face and spit in its eye. And you can't do that unless you have a great big, awesome God standing right at your side!"

WOW, that got my attention. Then I noticed how fast he was running and what a long and easy stride he had. All the anxious uncertainties (euphemism for fears) that every healthy young father has a right to have: career, financial security, masculine image, balance of time, and relationships, etc. didn't seem to bother him much either. He told me, "When I got cancer I figured some stuff out. Life is better now."

As I was writing this book, I was reading, David McCullough's, *1776*, about the American Revolution and came across Thomas Payne's article "The American Crisis." It opens with, "These are the times that try men's souls." I was struck by how these words resonate for someone facing cancer. Paine continues, "Tyranny, like hell, is not easily conquered; yet we have this consolation with us, that the harder the conflict, the more glorious the triumph. What we obtain too cheap, we esteem too lightly. Heaven knows how to set a proper price upon its goods; and it would be strange indeed, if so celestial an article as freedom should not be highly rated." [22] Freedom from the tyranny of fear, be it of a greedy English King or a slimy Dragon, is a precious thing well worth our pursuit.

Is it achievable for man on his own? Many would say it isn't. Little has a more clarion call to prayer than fear. There is nary a person who will not at least give it a shot. From what I know, prayer is not a cavalier undertaking. Oswald Chambers cautions us, "God is not some eternal blessing machine for man."[23] He is not a genie to put to work on our personal agenda.

Sharon, who had breast cancer, told me that one need not earn the right to be heard through righteous, rule abiding living or belonging to some church. Fortunately, God is not selective about who He listens or responds to. It is we who are selective in hearing what He has to say. If we can't or won't listen to Him, then it doesn't do much good to speak to Him in the first place. Patients that know Him tell me prayer to God, who is on call 24/7, is an amazing source of comfort when faced with fear.

Wendell, who had acute leukemia, told me, "Danger gets our attention. We go on full alert with whatever it takes to escape or overcome it. Thoughts about the leaking roof, the mortgage payment, and the next vacation are dropped, the slate is cleared and attention is riveted on the immediate threat. In that moment, Christ wants to enter in and grab our attention. He may bless us straightaway or He may want to teach us something first. The blessing may come later, even much later and often with a new understanding of what is really going on. However, if it is only the blessing one is looking for, the real message and the gift of understanding may be missed, and the real blessing may never come." Wendell was on a spiritual journey that clearly meant a lot to him and steadied his run.

In our next chapter we are going to power up the right foot of hope, but first, take action as suggested in this chapter.

- Focus only on what is knowable and necessary for today.
- Don't sacrifice today to what is uncertain in the future.
- Deciding on a plan and taking action to implement it decreases fear.
- Write down your plan, give it a timeframe, and start working on it. Then update it.
- Avoid fearful people. Don't give them any airtime; none at all.
- Beware of the Internet. It can confuse, mislead, and alarm you more than to help you.
- Consider talking to God about your fears.

Starting the Backstretch

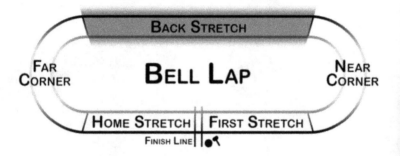

Chapter 12

Cultivate Hope – Power Up the Right Foot

"The joy in your heart rests on the peace in your soul, which stands on the strength of your hope."*24*

The backstretch starts with planting seeds of hope, cultivating them, then searching for ever better seeds, and cultivating them. This is really important because it is said that disappointment is the most common human emotion, meaning what you hoped for didn't come through for you. This is sadly an all too common experience for patients with cancer, but it need not be so. There are many things to hope for, some trivial and frivolous, others profound and essential. You must find and name them as there is nothing that fuels the strength to endure hardship like hope. Without it, physical strength and mental fortitude are worthless and rapidly defeated. So, it is essential to plant every seed of hope you can find and prospect for more.

Growing hope is like growing vegetables—fertilize, water, and cultivate. Nurturing hope is pretty easy, but good cultivation is a delicate task of identifying the weeds of false hopes, and pulling them out by the roots. Every gardener knows that weeds have deep roots and so do false hopes.

Just as weeds are drought resistant, false hopes are reason resistant. Weeds of false hope grow faster, often overshadowing the real ones. They may even flower and look attractive at first, before you discover their poison. They can consume your life faster than any cancer can consume your body.

Remember, illness is what happens to your life when disease attacks your body and controlling the illness is your responsibility. If you buy into something false, you're just expanding the ways the illness can hurt you. So, let's first focus on identifying the counterfeit hopes, the ones you get nothing for when you cash them in. Then you can cast them aside and focus your energy on the real ones that can bring you unfettered joy and will sustain you for the long run.

Identifying False Hopes

False hopes will come from well-meaning doctors, friends, family, and from deep within your own aching heart. The question is not whether they will appear, but whether you will recognize them as false. Even if you do, will you grab onto them anyway because you've nothing else better to grab? To avoid that, you need to find what is better so you can let go of what isn't, or resist grabbing on to it in the first place. Ask yourself, "What is false? How can it hurt and deceive me?"

There has never been a more hopeful time in cancer treatment medicine. We now understand more about how cancer cells behave, how to change their behavior, and how to kill them. Boutique cancer therapy that tailors treatment to each individual, optimizing efficacy, and minimizing toxicity was a dream yesterday and today a reality. However, it doesn't exist yet for every cancer and every person. The power of our research tools and the brilliance of today's investigators is absolutely mind boggling. New ideas are born every day and new treatments every year, but not yet for everyone.

All this good news doesn't really change the prognosis you have just been given which incorporates everything learned to date. Today, you are the benefactor of great past progress and the chance of further dramatic breakthroughs during your lifetime. However, the reality is the chance a miracle drug or any other treatment that will come along to dramatically change the prognosis for your disease is actually pretty small (if the progress of medicine in the last ten years is any indicator). Therefore, it is not worth calling it a big hope. Don't be fooled. Yes, it is a small hope, so put it in your hope chest, but look elsewhere for bigger ones.

False hope is like fool's gold. Fool's gold gets you excited at first, but when you take it to the bank they laugh at you. It is what people find when they are prospecting in the wrong place or when they don't really know what they're looking for. Once they have seen, held, and felt the real thing, they're not likely to be fooled again by an imposter.

Medical treatment for cancer is marvelous, but not perfect so better not be your sole basis for hope. At some point, usually when things are getting desperate, it disappoints you like a mirage. If that's the only hope you're standing on, you'll soon discover it is quicksand and you're going down—you just don't know when. Everyone who places all their hope in medicine knows this at some level and it doesn't feel good. They can feel the Dragon's breath. They have let it get too close.

I saw an advertisement the other day showing an exuberant woman with cancer recounting her meeting with a physician at an exalted medical center. She exuded, "The doctor said he had a plan for me, and another one after that. All I needed to hear from him was that there is hope." Doctors know what we all need and will cultivate your trust with hope every day that they can.

The question is what happens when they run out of good plans? Sooner, or later, most of them do. They often don't say so and people don't ask. One day they walk in and confess, "I'm out of tricks." Deep down everyone knows that day is coming. I could see it in their eyes and hear it in their voices. That is why early on we would, and you should, start cultivating a whole portfolio of other hopes that are not subject to the caprice of cancer and the limitations of research.

Beware of Family and Friends

You have just become a target for all kinds of well-meaning, smooth talking, unintentionally deceiving, and ever tempting "friends." They will come out of the woodwork, in the grocery store line, at the gym, across the back fence, and at church. They will be entirely sincere, but sincerity does not guarantee truth. The number of my patients waylaid by well-meaning neighborly advice is amazing. Many of those friends are captive to the very fears we have already been talking about. They are running madly in every direction away from their fears and beckoning you to follow. They would love to have your company

Some of the wild treatment ideas that will be offered will sound bizarre and others quite legitimate. Some individuals diversify their portfolio of hopes by adding all sorts of concoctions, diets, enemas, magnets or vitamins. That is not the kind of diversity I am encouraging. Those, when tried, feel good initially due to the hope inspiring placebo effect, an effect which is real, but short-lived because it never actually shrinks tumors or prolongs lives. You need something better.

For some the masquerade of the placebo effect lasts longer, but that is only for the folks who have slow-growing tumors where the very virtue of slow growth allows the pretense of placebo efficacy to go unexposed. Any situation where the cancer cannot be easily seen or measured nor experienced through painful symptoms is perfect to hide the falsity of a placebo's hope and can dissuade some from taking effective treatment. Meanwhile the cancer is free to grow unrecognized. Beware of well-meaning testimonials. One person's placebo does not make another's effective treatment.

Beware of Yourself

Some of the most subtle and deceptive false hopes are ones of our own making. They can seduce even the brightest and godliest. C.S. Lewis, a much respected Cambridge professor and Christian apologist, lamented, "What chokes every prayer and every hope is the memory of all the prayer Joy and I offered and all the false hopes we had. Not hopes raised merely by our own wishful thinking; hopes encouraged, even forced upon us, by false diagnoses, by x-ray photographs, by strange remissions, by one temporary recovery that might have ranked as a miracle. Step by step we were led up the garden path. Time after time, when He (God) seemed most gracious, He was really preparing the next torture."[25] These were the raw and real words of a man who loved God deeply, but had just lost his wife to breast cancer after having let himself be seduced by false hopes of his own making.

Joy Davidson was dying of breast cancer when C. S. Lewis married her and then she sustained a wonderful blessed remission. Then something happened for Lewis which I have seen happen too frequently to other Christians-both patients and families. They quite reasonably received the favorable turn of events as a blessing, in this case a remission from cancer. They were appropriately overjoyed and grateful. Then came the part where we all, in our humanity, seem so often to stumble. They attempted to ascribe their own hopeful understanding and expectations to the meaning and purposes of God.

When people do this, they almost invariably create false hope and, in so doing, they also create a trap for themselves. This happened to some acquaintances of my friend Wendell who had AML (Acute Myelogenous Leukemia). His miraculous remission was an answer to many prayers, but even as good and as long as it was, it wasn't the cure they came to expect. When the leukemia actually took his life, some were confused and others angry. It seems this time God had other plans.

Most often we remain blissfully blind to what we have done in grabbing on to a false hope. Other times, even before the trap is sprung, we start fearing that trouble is coming; we hear Dragon footsteps in the attic. Then we realize that we are not certain that the agenda we so hopefully ascribed to God may not really be indeed His. The Dragon is coming down the stairs, anxiety is creeping in, and peace is seeping away. When the trap is revealed, our agenda exposed, and the cure, the prolonged remission, the freedom from pain, the new happiness or harmony or whatever comes to naught, we get bewildered, maybe bitter, even deny that blessing ever occurred, and maybe even deny its source. The Dragon loves to deliver gifts of false hope because inside all the pretty wrapping is fear.

Wendell, a pastor, was concerned about all this. He cautioned, "Avoid this trap. Accept the blessing for all that it is for today, maybe an example of divine love or scientific brilliance, but don't add anything to it. Resist too much interpretation projecting what it means for the future. When mom makes your favorite dessert, you receive it with all the love intended. But when she doesn't make it every day thereafter, you don't conclude she has stopped loving you, or that the desert she made originally was a fluke."

Wendell went on, "In such events and in our response to them lays the essence of who God is and how little we understand. He does things to show us he loves us, but it is not the thing that is the love, nor is the pie. It is what is in the heart of the pie maker. If we have eyes only for the pie, we will miss the message and the messenger. Love is what we can count on Mom and God revealing to us over and over again in ways we can't always predict let alone prescribe. We may be able to hope for some, but we don't control any. The mystery remains mysterious and the pie is extra."

Another patient, Karen, seemed to know this. When her lymphoma unexpectedly responded again and dramatically to chemotherapy, she told me she was not going to stumble as C. S. Lewis had. She was going to enjoy and be grateful for this blessing in the present without making the joy and gratitude dependent on what might happen in the future. She told me she was confident that God loved her and that was enough. She wasn't going to second guess what was next; she didn't need to.

Beware of Denial or Bargaining Masquerading as Hope

There is a story I have repeatedly heard in a variety of iterations from patients or families. At the last minute, when all surgery, chemotherapy, radiation, and even bone marrow transplantation have failed, they feel their God has told them that He will heal them. Sometimes, they have added a gambit that such expectant faith will show how great God is and inspire others to the faith. Sadly, in every such situation I've witnessed, that kind of hope gambit has failed. Sadder still is that when that kind of hope fills a hope chest, there is neither room nor need for any other kind of hope. When it fails, they are hopeless, sometimes godless.

Poignantly, most of the people who are *being strong and* determined *to make it* in this situation know the gambit is of their own creation. The tone in their voices and the expressions on their faces betray a deeper understanding than they are willing to acknowledge. Desperation grows as the ignored writing-on-the-wall is transcribed into their lives. There it often creates a schism between loved ones, the miracle holdouts, and those just trying to say good-bye. The former shun the latter because of their *nonbelieving "negative energy"* and the much needed supportive interaction is impossible.

One of their desperate prayers is that they will not lose their faith, yet the peace that would be evidence of that faith is nowhere to be seen. I have seen lots of different kinds of divine miracles, but I have never seen a deathbed miracle where God sweeps in at the last moment, after all else has failed, to cure someone. I have seen no evidence that God plays games with us or tests us in that way. Hope for such a miracle is really no hope at all; it is fodder for the Dragon's deception.

Lasciate Ogne Speranza, Voi Chi'ntrate

In his allegorical poem, *Inferno*, Dante Alighieri and his pal Virgil glide beneath the inscription, "Abandon all hope, ye who enter here," as they pass through the gates of the underworld. The living who lack hope are already there. Just to avoid a living hell some choose a sterile, helpless, and hopeless resignation. They miss out on a lot.

Some are irreligious and others very religious. A medical school classmate of mine spent twenty-five years practicing and teaching cancer medicine at New York University. He had found himself working at times in pretty much a Jewish state, much as I had during my years a few blocks further north in Manhattan at The Mount Sinai Hospital. The majority of his patients were Jewish as were all of his associate physicians. If they themselves were not rabbis, then their local rabbi was frequently present and active in their healthcare. Struck as I had been with our new found abilities to lessen our patient's pain and misery during the last days and hours of their lives, my classmate had developed a palliative care team. He specialized in end of life decision-making and symptom control and was frequently called to interface with patients, their families, and their physicians.

At a recent reunion, he spoke despairingly of how challenging it was to care for some of the Orthodox community because, "They had no hope beyond this life, no sense of crossing the River Jordan, no promise of the land running with milk and honey, no promise of meaningful existence in Heaven—not until their messiah comes and the last trumpet sounds." Because of this, they would refuse palliative care and insist on aggressive investigations and treatments up to the last breath. Even if the patient or their family would "weaken," the Rabbi was there as a controlling presence to ensure it was done right. For a physician to be compassionately "too generous with morphine, or to fail to do every last futile x-ray, or to fail to give every last futile course of chemotherapy was to risk being fired."

It would seem that having no hope in neither a Messiah who has already come as professed by Christians nor His promises of Heaven can lead one to a hell on earth of endless treatment. It also demonstrates the ends to which some will go just to avoid being without the hope of a cure or remission. It sounds a word of caution ere any other of us fall in that trap. I have seen many similarly snared, but the choices that got them there seldom had anything to do with whether a Messiah has come or not, but everything to do with the Dragon.

Diversify Your Portfolio of Hopes

> *There are only two kinds of people, those who have dreams and those who had dreams!* – Gino Grunberg

Begin planting a whole garden of hope seedlings of many kinds and start watering them all. Hopes for today, hopes for tomorrow, next week, next month, and next year. Include little hopes and big hopes, like a visit to a place or person, some travel, some symptom improvement, some function regained, a celebration, a reunion, an event, a new project or the completion of an old one, a plan for baton passes, gifts, and on and on. Dream them up. Plan them. Schedule them. Don't let the fragility of one hope, like your hope for survival, keep you from dreaming up and pursuing all the others. However, you must hold them lightly and that's the hard part.

Ralph told me that the only way he could really savor a dream and hold it lightly was to have at least one dream/ hope that he could count on, and hold with all his strength. For him, that was his "foundational hope that Jesus is exactly who He says He is and His promises are exactly what He says they are." When Ralph did that, he found that his precarious hope for survival was less disabling and no longer prevented him from creating and pursuing all his other hopes.

He went on to instruct me that when he had a diversified portfolio of hopes, and one of them didn't come through, there were always others. He would share his hopes with God and invite God's creativity to inspire more. Ralph's confidence with that process uplifted him with the expectation that where one hope didn't play out another would; or if not, the greatest hope of them all always would. Ralph was at peace. That is rare among bell-lappers except among the Windrunners.

Seeking Windrunners' Peace:

- The joy in your heart rests on the peace in your soul, which stands on the strength of your hope.

- Just as weeds are drought resistant, false hopes are reason resistant.

- Weeds of false hope grow faster, often overshadowing the real ones.

- They may even flower and look attractive at first, before you discover their poison.

- They can consume your life faster than any cancer can consume your body.

- Therefore, ask yourself, "What is false? How can it hurt and deceive me?"

The Backstretch Journey

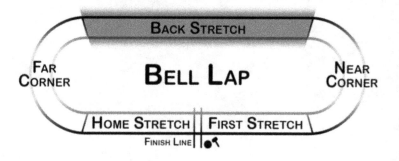

Chapter 13

Optimizing Your Basic Health

Now that you are catching your breath after all the intense complexities of the near corner, you are in remission, maybe off treatment or maybe on maintenance therapy and are settling into your new life's stride, it is time to pay attention to many things like relationships, goals, and dreams. However, general health habits and spiritual wellbeing are still primary. Your doctors have hopefully dealt with every system of your body from diet and dental care to your bowels, but one thing often over looked in the fray is your sleep. It is critical for your endurance, tolerance of therapy, memory, creativity, and enthusiasm. Most healthy people need 6-8 hours and when under stress they need even more sleep. The body does best with regularity. There are normal metabolic and hormonal functions which do better if you rise and retire at roughly the same time each day.

If you are young and healthy, you can abuse your body with an irregular lifestyle and get away with it, but with the biologic stresses of age and cancer treatment you will pay a price for poor eating habits and the lack of quality sleep: fatigue, poor memory, depression, decreased creative thinking, and more.

Fatigue is the number one side effect of chemotherapy. If potentiated by a poor night's sleep, it can defeat your ability to take effective treatment or live meaningfully during it. Taking a regular 10-20 minute power nap daily can be amazingly beneficial. Try to do it on a regular schedule. If you work, go to the car for lunch, and grab a quick one.

People under stress often find themselves awake for a couple hours around 3 a.m. with their brains bouncing from one concern to another. First, eliminate caffeine after 2 p.m., (some need to stop after noon) and back off on alcohol to one drink or less per night. While it can relax you and make you sleepy initially, later, after about 3 a.m. it can be stimulating and wake you up or give you that only half-asleep feeling.

If you find yourself exhausted without coffee as I did, you could have sleep apnea which can compromise anyone, but can be devastating for someone on treatment. It affects 25 percent of men and 10 percent of women irrespective of weight. Untreated, it can cause snoring, irritability, memory impairment, heart disease, and erectile dysfunction as well as depression, car accidents, job loss, and divorce. If there is any hint of this, get it checked out with an overnight sleep study.

The ability to fall asleep rapidly doesn't mean you are a great sleeper. It may signify a desperation for sleep even though you thought you slept soundly for 8 hours the night before. If you are one who is also desperate for coffee in the morning and repeatedly during the day or if you don't feel rested when you rise in the morning, it may be you were repeatedly stressed out during the night because sleep apnea stopped your breathing without your even knowing it. Sedatives and alcohol make it worse, but relatively simple things like sleeping on your side, oral devises, nasal dilators or a CPAP machine can give you your life back. It's not just about feeling good. It is about being able to take the most effective cancer treatment and taking care of your heart and other important organs. Coffee is great, but a good night's sleep is better.

Everything about cancer makes you tired: the diagnosis, the depression, the treatment, and the inactivity. A 2013 review of fifty-six studies on cancer related fatigue and exercise reported in the Harvard Men's Health Watch suggests, "Instead of resting, people with cancer related fatigue should try aerobic exercise if they can. This includes brisk walking, a light workout on a treadmill or exercise cycle, or water aerobics." Weight lifting was of no benefit against fatigue. In addition to the physical benefits, exercise improves sleep and lessons depression. Find someone to do it with and go for it. If you are lonely get a dog. It will love you as you deserve to be loved: unconditionally and become a great walking partner. Time is a wasting and everyone could use more love and energy. Incidentally, exercise helps keep the bowels moving, and helps everyone fall asleep. Just do it. Make a schedule and keep it.

Responding to the Motivation

Steve Jobs, founder and guru of Apple, told an audience at Stanford University, "Remembering that I'll be dead soon is the most important tool I've ever encountered to help me make the big choices in life. Because almost everything – all external expectations, all pride, all fear of embarrassment or failure – these things just fall away in the face of death, leaving only what is truly important!"[26]

The backstretch is about defining what is truly important in your life even if you're not planning to die soon, but particularly if you are. In horseracing, the backstretch is that part of the oval racetrack farthest from the spectators. It is the same for cancer patients. The entire crowd's attention garnered by the initial diagnosis and treatment is dwindling. Even the Dragon is slipping back in the shadows. The crowds that will line the home stretch are a long way off. This is a time just for you.

By now the acute shock of the diagnosis is subsiding, the time-consuming tests and confusing results are behind you, treatment has begun bringing hope and some reassurance to all, denial and bargaining have hopefully been abandoned, the faces of your fears identified, and you are prospecting for realistic hopes to invigorate each new day. It is time for a new strategy for the rest of your life and to position yourself for the baton pass in the far corner.

Long-distance runners think of their races in terms of critical zones and cruising zones. For you, the near corner and the home stretch are critical zones where unpredictable challenges are coming at you rapid fire. The backstretch is a comfort zone where you can lengthen your stride and cruise. However, it still has an essential agenda which, if ignored or wasted in denial or trivial pursuits, will lead to a worthless far corner and a crash on the home stretch. Nobody likes to think about the far corner or homestretch, but because they are out there somewhere you will do best if you do a little preparing for them now. Size them up and mull them over while you have lots of time to do so.

If you ran well in the near corner, you no longer need to keep mixing it up with your adversaries fighting for the inside lane and your heart. You can swing out wide where you can spend some time alone and do some thinking. If cancer has torn the cover off of life to reveal emptiness inside, now is the time you have to do something about that. From the new vantage point, look at life and figure out what really matters to you.

Look over at the misery of those in the pack who are still running the rat race, fighting for the fast lane, tripping over denial of all kinds of issues they have refused to admit, and are boxed in by all kinds of fears they are too blind to see. Some of them are using their job or their manufactured identity to escape their responsibilities as a person, a parent, a spouse, a brother/sister, a daughter/son. You have to let your cancer strip away the superficialities and start searching for the essentials. Let it be the worst that reveals the best, then your actions will define your personhood with substance and character.

Experiencing the Freedom to Discover

It can feel lonely in the outside lane running a different race than the crowd. You alone have cancer and you alone have a future that is in limbo. Compassionate friends are wonderful, but you are still alone. If compassion fatigue sets in and they pull back, you can feel even more alone. The thinking you need to do, you need to do alone, so take advantage of this time and focus your thoughts. Real is not how you were born, it is what you become. It takes time in the workshop with cutting and hammering, taking apart and putting back together, and letting go and grabbing on.

What you've done with your life may have brought success, but it is *who* you have become and are becoming that brings significance and that is what counts; that is what they will remember! The doing may have brought worldly applause, but it soon fades and is forgotten. Your *being,* however, can send a message that extends through the next generation and beyond. The backstretch is your last chance to complete who you are becoming and the far corner is your last chance to show them how you did it. It is also where you show them how the answers to life's big questions, the ones seldom considered until the backstretch, have made a difference.

Your Spiritual Journey

You can do what so many of my patients surprised themselves by doing, i.e., going on a spiritual journey, many for the first time, others to resume a journey once abandoned. Those journeys have taken them in a variety of directions, often with a few twists and turns along the way. Some journeys have been more intriguing than others, some more durable, but almost all are meaningful.

Most importantly, the journey got each of them engaged in asking the big questions.

Who am I really?

Why am I here?

What is the purpose of the rest of my life in spite of cancer?

If God really exists, does He have a role here?

What might that be?

Did I ever go wrong along the way, and, if so, where?

Is there anything I wish I had done differently?

Is there anyone I've disappointed or hurt?

Is there any relationship I could've handled better?

Is there anything I can do now to make amends?

Not easy stuff, but strip away your pride and do it anyway; get real. No one is watching except maybe God (if He is up there). And if He is, God already knows it all anyway and is just waiting for you to figure it out. If indeed He is, then He is just waiting to replace any burden of regret or shame you've got with forgiveness and any confusion with insight. That is, if you choose to ask.

The wounded need courage to find a counselor to uncover their scars and help heal them. Often, the deepest wounds have come from family right out of childhood or adolescence, others from peers or partners. Wounds all start to bleed when the stress of cancer picks at them. Address them now and unburden yourself so you can fight the cancer better.

No one I know who has chosen to do a personal inventory of their life and let it guide them on their journey has regretted it. Sometimes it leads to a forgiveness fest for you and others, and when it is done, it lightens their load as well as yours and adds spring to everyone's stride. Sometimes it brings inspiration, new hope, and new energy to run faster and often longer than we ever expect.

The Windrunners were all journeyers. When you decide what direction your journey will take, find a fellow traveler, a friend or a mentor, or someone on the track ahead of you. While you're at it, get out the bucket list you made in the first stretch and start punching it. Be intentional about both the journey and the list, and schedule them. Remember, memories of what you have done are not nearly as good as hopes of what you will do. Perhaps, the journey will reveal hopes that disease and time cannot erase.

Many find that first thing in the morning is a great journey time for reading, reflecting, and journaling. Try it. Make it a habit. As this time comes to an end, focus on the very day that is before you, on the precious present, and what you can do with it. Never let what is impossible corrupt what is.

"Mindfulness means paying attention in a particular way, on purpose, in the present moment," writes Jon Kabat-Zinn. [27] Some find his thoughts helpful in their quest for physical and spiritual healing. One advocate who found meditation very helpful described it to me as sort of like prayer, but directed inward toward his own mind. His wife agreed, but countered that its limitation was that it left success all up to him, whereas prayer for her recruited divine power to guide and intercede in her thoughts, relationships, and the biology of her body. Her experience was that prayer provided for her a peace that continued even when she was too tired to pray or meditate. She found comfort in believing it was not all up to her. Clearly they are on a journey together. It will be fascinating to speak to them in a few years.

Figure out what part of the day and week provide the most free time and energy for punching your bucket list. Then be aggressive in your scheduling, and adjust as needed. Get on with it. Do it now. Don't let indecision or uncertainty fritter your life away.

Optimizing Your Basic Health

- First thing in the morning is a great time for reading, reflecting, and journaling. Try making it a habit.
- As meditation time comes to an end, focus on the very day that is before you, on the precious present, and what you can do with it.
- Never let what is impossible corrupt what is.
- Then begin to ask yourself the big questions in preparation for the baton pass:

  Who am I really?

  Why am I here?

  What is the purpose of the rest of my life?

  If God really exists, does He have a role here?

  What might that be?

  Did I ever go wrong along the way, and, if so, where?

  Is there anything I wish I had done differently?

  Is there anyone I've disappointed or hurt?

  Is there any relationship I could've handled better?

  Is there anything I can do now to make amends?

  Who will I pass the baton to, when, and what?

Chapter 14

Planning the Baton Pass

The baton is truth, but it is more than the facts of life and the laws of science, more than the lessons of history and religion. It is your truth, all the wisdom you have accumulated, some from your parents, some from your studies, and some painfully through years of interaction with the physical and spiritual world. It is a treasure which cost you a lifetime to accrue and for which you are the steward until it is passed along to the next generation.

A Strategy for Young and Unready

The heart wrenching poignancy of a parent dying before their children are grown and married may be unavoidable, but the tragedy of that parent disappearing from a child's heart and memory is. When you cannot finish your parenting in person, you must find another way. Sometimes, it's easier to write things than to say them especially if the kids are too young to understand. By writing, you create an indelible message that can be revisited through the years over and over at any time day or night. Some write a book pouring out their heart and wisdom to those they leave behind. Others write each child, sibling, and spouse a love letter full of affirmation and encouragement. Decide what you want to do and start. It is never too soon. You don't want to find yourself on the homestretch dragging a chain of shoulda, coulda, wouldas behind you. Even more important than preparing advice for your kids for their future is showing them how to cope with the present as it unfolds, how to deal with the tuff stuff, and how to find a silver thread, something good, something positive, and how to always focus on it.

Deciding when and how much of your cancer story to share with your kids is always hard. Just remember that if you choose to hide the truth you cannot hide your feelings. Kids invariably sense them and when they don't know where they come from they feel even worse. Try to share as much as you can of the truth as often as you can to help them make sense of it and process their feelings. When you share your honest feelings about the illness, you are modeling vulnerability and honesty, and inviting them to do the same. They will be healthier in the long run and you will be less anxious. They will all face difficulties someday. Protecting them now will not prepare them for tomorrow. They likely live in an illusion of safety which is now shattering. You have a rare opportunity to show them how to find the pieces and start putting them back together into something that can be good. It will take time, but teaching them how to do it is essential.

There are times when the intended recipient isn't physically present, emotionally mature or spiritually receptive enough. Yet, there is the hope that more years of living will bring them to a place of readiness. So, many will write, planning for their words to be read six months, a year or many years later like on key birthdays (16, 21, 40) or on the eve of a marriage, year three or four when infatuation is fading, or at the birth of a child. These letters often described the writer's own experiences at those ages and pass on bits of advice that would be given, if only they could be there.

Open for the kids a window into the things that helped you become you. Tell them about your favorite books from each season of your life and why you loved them, about your favorite music and special experiences that go with it, and your favorite places to visit and how they moved you. Share about challenging situations and how you made the hard decisions. Tell them about significant people and special friends and how they influenced you. They need to know where your passions came from, what and who inspired them, and who wounded or nurtured them.

Pictures are particularly important. Take or find pictures of you being you, especially your expressions and especially you with your kids. Not the documentary posed shots, but the impromptu ones where you are engaging with them, tickling, hugging, wrestling, and adoring. Do it with a video camera if you can and capture your voice and your laughter. Long after spoken words are forgotten, kids have got to be able to look back and *see* how much you loved them. You can even put together a treasure trove of quotations, mottos, scriptures, and pictures. Frame some to hang or sit on a bedside table.

Create confidence by bestowing it. Write individually or collectively to your kids, the young and old alike, commissioning them with responsibilities, both in the near future and down the road. Tell them what you expect a big brother to do for the younger ones and vice versa. Tell them how you're counting on them to love and care for their mother/dad when you no longer can, and how they might best do that. Be specific, and while you are at it, teach them about the different languages of love: quality time together, words of affection and affirmation, deeds of service, gifts, and hugs. They need to know how to take care of each other in every way they can.

Check out www.mychapters.org. This site is designed to encourage and provide hope for cancer patients. It also provides an app to chronicle and preserve for the generations to come a patient's voice, personality, and legacy. The app is projected to be available early 2016. It enables a patient to setup a "Private Time Capsule" with privacy settings and with multiple sub capsules for use by friends and family so each can chronicle/write about life's journey. They can add history, feelings, wisdom, and accolades, as well as pictures and videos. It can then be opened daily for encouragement or later as a message from the past to the future.

Create a Measure of Your Own Peace

Carl professed no fear of death, but a terrible fear of being forgotten. He feared that in the end, his life would not have really mattered. He confided that his worst fear was that he would drop the baton and die with regrets. He was a man of few words, but a big heart. His family was so scattered and distant that few could afford to visit him and he was beyond traveling. He knew he couldn't call them and be able to say what he wanted to say; there was just too much.

He had not put pen to paper for over fifty years, but writing became his sanctuary. He wrote a letter to his whole family with special addendums for each. He spent all of the few months he had composing his letter. It became a focus for each day and the priceless core purpose of his backstretch.

Dying was a pretty solitary experience for Carl, as it is for many, made worse by neither knowing how much time he had left nor when to call the kids to his side for a last good-bye. Suddenly death stared him in the face, but he was ready. The anxiety had left him. His message was secure on paper where he left it on the kitchen table for them to find.

As it turned out, a few of the kids arrived at the hospital just before the end. He had his thoughts already collected and was able to deliver many more of them than he had ever imagined. Anxiety was gone and a kind of joy like a poultice entered his room. By taking control of transmitting his legacy in writing, this fretful but caring man had created a measure of his own peace.

Project Your Parenting into the Future

Gretchen attacked her high grade, but Stage 3 breast cancer like a quarterback. She rallied her extended family as support staff, recruiting her kids to take on all kinds of new responsibilities so that she could focus all of her energy on an aggressive treatment program of chemotherapy, that life-prolonging poison and marvel of our modern world aimed at curing her. We all cheered when she completed a grueling six-month course and started getting back into shape to resume her life. We all cried three years later when she relapsed. She went after her treatment again and with zeal, but clearly hearing the bell ringing, she focused her zeal differently.

Accepting the sad fact that relapsed breast cancer is never cured, she chose treatments having the least side effects rather than the highest response rates. Then she focused on being the best mother as long as she could. Recognizing that she was destined to die before her daughters would become women, she had her husband take a video of her speaking directly into the camera advising her daughters on how their little bodies would change as they reach puberty and the social challenges they would experience at that time and about boys.

Then she recorded another segment for her daughters to see when they were contemplating marriage and another for just before the first child's birth. Before each segment Gretchen would record a vignette of their life together as mother and daughters revealing just how much she had loved and enjoyed each one, how she would be looking down from heaven and waiting until they would meet again.

My family has just done something similar for my ninety-year-old father. He is not dying, but we chose to do a composite family history/eulogy to celebrate his life while he is still with us and to create an almost living memory for the grandkids that will never really get a chance to know him. We collated pictures from each of our albums and snatched segments of old family movies Mom had taken. Then we recorded each sibling recounting a special memory to capture their perspective and also their voices. We also recruited a friend, Chris Ballasiotes,[28] to come over with his movie camera to record dad answering a series of interview questions: memories of his childhood and parents, silly things he recalled about each of us as kids, things he loved about Mom, meaningful things about his life's work as a physician, what things he would've done differently given the chance, and his advice for each of us for years to come.

Then we gave him our old beat up copy of *Uncle Remus* and had him read about Brer Rabbit, Brer Fox, and Brer Bear using all those funny, made up voices he had used for each of the characters when we were kids. We videoed him walking around our home with his steadfast companion, Barney, an aging golden retriever, and captured him stealing kisses from daughters and granddaughters. Siblings' words were spliced over the pictures and video, and then music of his era was added. A copy went to all the kids, grandkids, nephews, and nieces. I regret we didn't capture Mom in the same way during her year-long struggle with lung cancer. The project was great fun for Dad and it compelled me to spend focused time with him that I will always treasure.

Many of the elderly with waning mental faculties fall into silence unable to participate in conversations regarding current events with the younger set, but distant memories are often so intact that they can avidly engage in wonderful reminiscing once given the chance. Now, we all celebrate Dad by watching the video together at Christmas time. He watches it again and again whenever he gets lonely or when he wants to see those old black and white images of Mom smiling and laughing–just being Mom and his sweetheart.

Create a Partnership with the Generations to Come

All of these writings, pictures, voice recordings, and videos create a "partnership of the generations between those who are living, those who have passed and those who are yet to be born"[29] If you do these things, you can start living forever right now. As *The Gladiator*, Maximus Decimus Maridius, inspired his legions, "What we do here today will echo in eternity."[30] If you pass the baton well, it will resound through the generations.

So, tell your story and tell it again. Emphasize what you have learned. Tell them where the shoals were, what rocks you have hit, and what storms you have weathered. These are the stories of truth and experience that are the real treasures. Tell them your favorite movies and books and they will always think of you when they encounter them. In a small way, they will understand what created you and is now part of them, and what enabled you to love the way you loved calling them to do the same. It will inspire them to pursue their passions as you pursued yours.

Chance and circumstance manipulate our lives often in ways unbidden, but it is up to us and to us alone to choose the attitudes with which we embrace such misfortune. Those attitudes display more meaning than words and are far more indelible. Know that the kids are often watching more closely than they are listening and don't miss any opportunity to show them how to live in the face of adversity including cancer.

Do you ever wonder what stories your grandparents' bones could tell, what treasures went to the grave, now out of your reach, that might have informed or even changed your life? Grandpa and Grandma paid for them dearly, but they are forever lost and now you are paying for them with your blood, sweat, and tears. Will your grandchildren stand on your shoulders as they engage their worlds or will they stand foot to dirt because you were too disinterested or sidetracked on a backstretch of glory and hedonism and ignored your chance to write the prologue to their next chapter in the family story?

Some of what you learn as you write will be great fodder for conversations you will have with the curious and caring people who ask, "How are you?" Most of them don't have a clue how to respond if you give them the real nitty-gritty answer about your cancer and if you give it to them, will be so uncomfortable as to avoid you in the future. But if you are able to engage them with, "Here is something this cancer experience has got me thinking about...," or, "This is what I have been learning," or "Now I understand what grandma was trying to say when...," then little by little you pass bits of the baton to many people because they always open the door with that question and your response won't frighten them away. Indeed, they may come back for more.

Secrets

It is the time for telling secrets that have held you or others prisoner. It is a time to come out of any "cage of guilt"[31] created at first by a little lie or deceptive omission, but then perpetuated by more lies to protect the first which made the bars bigger and bigger. It is not just about breakout freedom or divine forgiveness, but it is "so that the person you're confessing to knows that they're not alone."[32] Small lies and omissions are common in life, but they seldom forecast the entrapment they create. When a mentor confesses, they not only break themselves free, but they also model how confession and authenticity enable relationships to grow and individuals to thrive. Find them, even if they seem small and white, and boldly wash them away.

Before you decide to tell the secret you have been harboring, you must consider why you would do so. If it is just to purge yourself of guilt but may cause harm of any kind, you must reconsider your plan. The coming clean should be healing and never destructive of a relationship. Keep your focus on the endgame which hopefully isn't about your own relief of guilt, but the healthy growth and healing of someone you care about.

You can open the topic with something like "I regret I didn't have the courage to tell the whole story years ago, or that I withheld the parts that I was ashamed of, or I regret I was more concerned about my reputation and what people thought of me than I was about you and ..."

Be careful with both your secrets and your accomplishments. You don't want to harm or create a burden with either one. The issue with secrets is obvious, but less so with achievements. The word legacy conjures up visions of grandeur, material provision, and a litany of successful endeavors in athletics, business, parenting, creativity or civic service. Beware, the first casualty of success can be humility. Don't let it happen.

For most heroes in real life, that is not the case. Their greatest treasures are healthy loving relationships. So, inspire children with your achievements, but measure your net worth in terms of quality relationships, something possible for everyone irrespective of wealth, physique, talent or intellect.

Many children are wounded by their parent's legendary legacy of either achievement or dissipation, as if a script has been written with their lives and is either unattainable or dreadfully possible. So, always leave your audience with a vision for what is both good and also possible. It is not a time for critique.

Remember, words of anger or unforgiveness uttered before death last forever.

Kids who were starved for affection and affirmation can become either very good parents, knowing full well what they didn't get and will be sure to give, or they can become crippled people-pleasers, unable to assert themselves with voice or deed in dysfunctional marriages and unsatisfying jobs. If you recognize any shortcoming in your parenting, the power and opportunity to heal is still yours as long as you are.

I am told that relationships are the only things that survive the grave and that all the love you created here will be there also. For the Heaven bound there will be a grand reunion, but only after a sit-down talk with God at Heaven's Gate when He will ask, "How did you do with those children I entrusted to you?" If there is anything you can do to mend or improve those relationships, you may as well do it now and start savoring the results–and save yourself some embarrassment at the gate when the Voice From Above says, "Take a seat, let's have a talk."

Planning the Baton Pass

- Tell your story often and tell it again.
- Emphasize what you have learned.
- Tell them where the shoals were, what rocks you have hit, and what storms you have weathered.
- These are the stories of truth and experience that are the real treasures.

The Far Corner

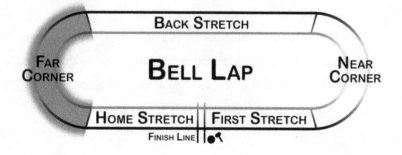

The Far Corner starts when your first relapse occurs. For the vast majority of cancer patients, this means cure is no longer possible. Another remission may be possible, but in all likelihood it will not be as long as the first; perhaps half as long, maybe less. With each relapse the likelihood of subsequent remission becomes less likely and shorter. So, if with the wisdom you have gained down the back-stretch and you have anything left in your life you want to complete, it is time to get on with it. If you are blessed with another remission or more time than you need, you can do it all over again.

Chapter 15

Pass the Baton

"We know that every moment is a moment of grace, every hour an offering; not to share them would to mean to betray them. Our lives no longer belong to us alone, they belong to all those who need us desperately."[33] (Élie Weisel)

"If you don't pass the baton, they may as well bury you in shallow nameless grave, because you will be soon forgotten." ("Dropped Batons Spell Disaster for US Relay Teams," Sports News Headline, Beijing, 2008)

The 4 X 100 meter relay is a premier Olympic track event in which six four-member teams compete on an oval track. Each of the four runners on a team completes 100 meters in a prescribed order, each carrying the relay baton, a 12-inch cylindrical stick, their segment of the race and then when exhausted and totally spent, skillfully pass it within a 20-meter changeover box to their next teammate. It is the responsibility of the incoming runner to thrust the baton into the outstretched hand of the outgoing runner who never looks back. "Polished handovers can compensate for a lack of basic speed to some extent and disqualifications for dropping the baton or failing to transfer it... are common." (Wikipedia)

You already know that illness is what happens to your life as disease affects your body and that an intentional strategy is necessary to overcome it. Because relapse confirms that your cancer is incurable (occasional exceptions: lymphoma, acute leukemia and testicular cancers), it's time for the next phase in your strategy. It is also time to look over your shoulder for the Dragon in disguise who will be coming after you with new fears and new invitations from denial.

You have just entered the far corner and it's time for the final baton pass. No one can tell you how long the corner will last or whether there will be more remissions. They can only tell you that the chances for more remissions are less likely and will be shorter. So, it is time to be serious about running the far corner well, accelerate your pace, and pass the baton.

In life, it is only the *person we are* that competes with the *person we could become*. One can do a lot of catch-up in a meaningful backstretch, and a polished handover to make up for past missed opportunities, like the ones you never saw until they had blown by.

Gail Devers, three-time Olympic gold medalist, gives advice for success: "The key is the outgoing runner is responsible to give a good target and incoming runner must have the eyes to look for that target and put that baton in there." Some of us will be lucky enough to have kids who plant themselves at our feet eager for what we have to say, but if they don't, we must have "eyes for the target." It's not up to us whether they hang on to it, but it is up to us to stick the pass, to find them, set the stage, wash it with confession or forgiveness as needed, create the moment, and pass the baton.

Do it One-on-One

One-on-one times are often best for the ticklish or tender stuff. I am not dying, but I do have a stent in a coronary artery and could croak in the mountains while the terrain is pushing my limits. So, whenever I get a chance I pass the baton. One autumn evening at sunset, I found myself sitting on a mountaintop with one of my unmarried sons. It was a perfect time for baton passing in the middle of which he popped the question, "Dad, how about the sex talk?" So, we had it, along with how to love, romance, and care for a wife in marriage. It was precious and would have never happened at the family dinner table or over coffee, though maybe over a beer. Create those one-on-one opportunities and it will happen.

The bell lap baton pass is not a one-time, one person event limited to the far corner. The backstretch is about preparing oneself for the final passes in the last corner, but you can start passing batons of wisdom as soon as you're ready. The final batons are the most precious words of truth, vision, and blessing, culled out, distilled down, and delivered on a silver platter. You want to be sure you get them right, so the early backstretch is about searching for, thinking through, living out, and validating the gems to pass on. Translate your failures into warnings, your successes in to significance, and launch all those you care about into their future off your shoulders.

You cannot control whether others will remember your story, but if you write the last chapter well coming through the far corner, the chances are good. You can reach beyond the next generation if you show them as well as tell them how it's done. The far corner gives you a unique platform, so speak from it. The only question is whether you have something worth saying. It is certain that if the message you speak and live is, "It's all about wonderful me," the audience will lose attention rapidly.

There are valuable things you can teach with words, but the most important things you have to show are your passion, your creativity, and your truth. If you love your wife, trust your God, care for the less fortunate, believe in hard work, accept responsibility, you have to show it. There is no more powerful time to do that than when you're rounding the corner into the home stretch, and only when necessary use words.

Stick the Pass

As Gail Devers sprinted into the changeover box, she would yell "stick hand" and slap the baton into the back reaching handoff teammate, and not let go until it was pulled out of her hand. That is what you've got to do. Be sure the messages get passed. If it is forgiveness, don't mince words. Stick it, get it out, and follow it with a hug. If it is love, say it with your whole body. If it is teaching, show them how it is done.

Annabelle was a delightful old fashion grandma with breast cancer who, on her bell lap, took her granddaughter into the kitchen and said in her lilting southern drawl, "Darlin', today I am gonna teach you how to make my fried chicken, then tomorrow it's going to be my Chocolate Bundt Cake. Your mother's never goin' to do it. Cooking isn't her thing."

Nona was an ever cheerful Greek widow also with breast cancer who, when she heard the bell, announced to her big sons, "It's time to teach you how to make my baklava." She did and for years thereafter those two men would bring into our office the baklava they had made and we would all celebrate their mother.

There was Anne, a spirited Italian woman from the old country with a swarthy olive complexion, a sun ripened face animated with wrinkles, and hands made strong by a life of tilling the earth and milking cows. She had already lost her husband, and her grown son was too far-off to receive a mother's baton. I think she decided I was to become the one to whom to pass on her love of food and wine.

She would often invite me to her home where she would walk me through her gardens naming the plants and tasting herbs fresh from the cutting. She gave me starts for tomatoes, parsley, sage, and basil always instructing how to plant and care for them. We would sit in the afternoon sun under her grape arbor sipping her homemade wine and nibbling on all kinds of things from her kitchen savored with garlic she had grown and drenched in olive oil she had pressed. Before breast cancer consumed her, she gave me her corks, sieves, and barrels along with instructions on how to make her fruit wines. Although the barrels still sit empty in my cellar, they are full of memories of her passion for food and friendship.

Then there was Bill. He took his sons and grandsons on a mock Montana cattle roundup where they would camp out in the open and saddle up before dawn. He wanted them to experience the crisp dewy mountain air and a magenta sunrise as they rode out to roust the cattle. That had been an indelible part of his youth and his story, and he wanted to be sure it got passed on first-hand. He started planning the trip when he hit the backstretch, and pulled it off just before the far corner. They all savored it over and over again as they celebrated him down the home stretch.

There was also Mark. He bought an old car to rebuild with his son just as he had with his dad back in the hot-rodding days of the '50s. He didn't tell his son who they were building it for or why. The son didn't even know that his dad had heard the bell, but he reveled in the dedicated dad-time. He learned how to weld, to tune a carburetor, rebuild a starting motor, and plane a head. When Bill became too weak to work, he would sit in the garage and tell his son what to do, and they talked about all kinds of things, the things men only talk about when they are grubbing in the shop, sweating in the woods or sharing a brew.

Mark had no choice but to quit working as the cancer grew, but he did have a choice what to do with his new-found free time and he chose to spend a chunk of it passing the baton to his son. Those were getting-real times, happy times, the kind you cannot buy, that financial security doesn't guarantee, and selfishness and easy living cannot create. It was the happiness that comes only when you give something of yourself that matters.

One of my favorites was Fred. He had earned his living in manufacturing and maintenance, and he knew how to fix anything. His cancer caused too much back pain for him to do physical things with his son. Also, his son was too busy with his own important job to find the time for dad, so Fred found another way to pass the baton that overcame those two obstacles. He read stories to his grandkids, many from the Bible as well as fairy tales and adventures. He got his arms around them again and again, and truths beyond words passed to those little kids. His daughter and daughter-in-law worked out a schedule to bring one or two of the grandkids over two or three times a week to listen to grandpa read, and sometimes the moms would skip their errands just to sit around the corner to listen and remember.

These stories may sound rather storybook romantic and they always are when people get real and loving. Create your own.

Go Beyond Tradition

Passing the baton is an elaboration of an age-old deathbed tradition of uttering a few final words before the body's long nap in the dirt, but it can be much more. The book of Genesis recounts how the blind and dying patriarch, Isaac, called his first-born, Esau, to his bedside to bestow his blessing. Generations later, Joseph took his two sons to the bedside of their dying grandfather, Jacob, to receive his blessing. Jacob called his twelve sons to his bedside to give them final instructions about inheritance and responsibilities.

To this day, there is a part of Jewish tradition that ritualizes deathbed repentance, confession, ordering of family affairs, instructions for life, and blessings. That is a wonderful practice, but passing the baton can be even more especially when started early. There are as many ways to pass it as there are people to do it. Find yours. It doesn't take money or skill, just a willing and motivated heart. Get on with it.

Don't postpone it to those waning deathbed hours. If you do, it is unlikely that much will ever happen and your descendants will be much the poorer. It is too important to be relegated to the last slot on your dance card when disease and medication-induced delirium can all too easily steal your thoughts and even your ability to speak. Even if you are in full possession of your faculties, courage can wane and sorrows defeat the best intentions.

Plan Ahead and be Intentional

The baton-pass needs to be planned in the backstretch, then executed with words in the far corner, and reinforced with your life throughout. The homestretch should be left entirely for applause. Clearly those seduced by fear and denial never get to the backstretch or make a good handoff and that is why the Dragon keeps throwing them to you.

Few can boast of perfect lives; we have made too many mistakes, but we can all run great bell laps worthy of cheers on the homestretch. Remember the song about rain coming down on a sunny day? That's what the homestretch can be like, a flood of tears shared by all those thankful and hopeful people that are cheering for you on every heavy step approaching Heaven's Gate.

We all bring a cultural legacy of how the end-of-life comes about. It is a conglomerate of all the deaths we have witnessed either at the bedside or in the movies. Those legacies become your unconscious script until you write another. When you do, it can become part of the script of everyone around you, perhaps even the dominant one. If you do it well, there will be no need for a rewrite.

That is what this book is about: how to do just that. If you were my patient, I would covenant with you to care for you as best as I am able and I would charge you with passing your baton. Trust us at the cancer center to do everything humanly possible to extend the length and quality of your life, while you discover and pursue the purpose for which you're lucky enough to have a bell lap. We will beat back the disease while you outwit the Dragon. We will coach you, but you have to do the running.

It's not about duty, it's about opportunity. It is not about strapping another "to do" list on your already weary back, but an opportunity to prepare a final gift of words for those who desperately need to hear them.

Wounds that may Never Heal

Walking the hospital halls with family members after a death, I have heard a litany of accolades, but also sad disappointments usually from those who had waited for, but not received, some resolution or healing of a relationship. The unfortunate ones usually started with what seemed to be obligatory charitable words of hollow praise for the departed, and then launched into bitterness because of the wounds that mother or father had caused years before. So often there were disappointments that could have been healed by heartfelt words of understanding or forgiveness that would not have erased the past deeds, but would have limited or eliminated the repercussions. Don't let this happen. Don't go to your grave with any unresolved, unforgiven or un-repented words tattooed on your soul, or theirs.

Sometimes there were subliminal messages from a dying parent that would become festering wounds that could play out in their children's live for years or become the work for tomorrow's counselors. So many of those could have been lessened by a parent who communicated their own struggles and confessed their own weaknesses, but in the end, in spite of them, held out loving arms. Even after many years, I keep hearing of the pain of the unresolved wreckage of past relationships with the departed.

Father Wounds

When you spend time around a group of men, sooner or later, someone will speak about their father. They will tell a story about him, the importance of his words, elbow to elbow mentoring, and how it all influenced who they have become. One after another will speak up, but then there will be those who remain silent.

When they begin to speak, it is either with anger or tears. Their stories of pain and the aftermath of a failed father relationship are so common that they could be reading from the same script. "I never heard my dad say he loved me. I felt like nothing but a tax deduction. If I got a 3.0 GPA, it decreased his risk of having to support me, but I never got an 'atta boy. I became an affirmation junkie and am to this day. Now it is like a duty I place on the shoulders of those around me to meet my desperate needs for approval."

Then another, "Despite how hard I tried, my father always had other champions. I was okay with not being a star, but he wasn't!" Or, "In the Japanese culture, kids try to make their parents proud. That's hard when your parent's interests are different than your own. I just wasn't equipped to be like them, so I could not succeed in their eyes. It was horrible to always feel not good enough. Although I'm highly successful in my own field, not-good-enough is how I feel deep down inside."

Another would say, "Dad didn't put his arm around me and tell me, 'Here is where we are going. This is what it is all about. Here is the big picture.' Everything I learned, I learned on my own. I was an orphan."

Then an angry one who was no longer angry speaks up, "My dad was mean as hell when I was a kid. He didn't talk to me much, but he beat me a lot. I hated him, but after years apart I discovered that time had mellowed him. When he finally let me into the depths of his life, I learned how hard his childhood had been and how stressful and confusing it had been trying to make a living, raise a family, and be a dad. I found myself feeling compassion for him. Now, my anger and resentment are almost gone as I work on the process of forgiving him. It has taken some time, but we're almost friends now."

When the revered Green Bay Packers and Minnesota Vikings quarterback, Brett Favre, lost his father, he realized that he had spent his whole career trying to prove himself to him. "I knew he was proud of me, but he was one of those who never said it. He never said it to me."

The elder Favre had driven his son relentlessly even after Brett reached the NFL and became the holder of virtually every significant NFL passing record, and winner of three MVP awards. His dad was a great man, savvy coach, and Brett's biggest fan, but he was always critical. Brett was reminded, "You're only as good as your last pass." With missed passes, he was rewarded by, "You couldn't hit a bull in the ass with a bass fiddle today." When Irv died, Brett said, "I thought it was a relief." Even the years that followed were filled with, "lingering insecurity." "There was always this little man on my shoulder pad saying 'prove you can do this'." Lousy bell lap, Irv. You left wounds.

However, I bet Irv had a story of his own wounds, most likely from his father. One could speculate that there was no loving mutual understanding and acceptance when death separated them either. Wounds get passed from generation to generation as well as wisdom, and probably a lot easier. It doesn't need to be that way.

Manipulation is a handy parental tactic, sometimes necessary for child safety and motivation, but when it becomes self-serving for a parent's agenda or identity needs, it can become destructive and leave wounds that putrefy. For those parents mellowed by years of living who can give up their need for control, it is time to go back, rethink, and undo whatever they can for the sake of their children and grandchildren. Too often, guilt or shame can keep us from going back and mending those fences broken down during the earlier, blind power years. Shuck those two and get on with the mending.

Your Story Is for Teaching

Your story is not your own. It is meant to be shared for good. None is too weird, too shameful or too tragic, but that it can reveal valuable truths. None deserves to be buried and forgotten. Each tells of the odd ebb and flow of hope and heartache, choice and consequence. They are all the intensely personal pieces to life's puzzle that we're all trying to solve. While not meant for everyone, they are meant for someone for whom they will have special meaning. Offer your story as a gift. The recipients will become its custodian, and in time they will blend and preserve it with their own, and pass it on.

With his driving cadences and plaintive refrains, Credence Clearwater, delivered a sad message and a poignant plea to the '60s generation that is every bit as apt today:

"The first thing I remember, was asking Papa, why
For there were many things I didn't know.
And daddy always smiled and took me by the hand
Saying, someday you'll understand.

Well, I'm here to tell you now, each and every mother's son
That you'd better learn it fast, you'd better learn it young,
'Cause someday never comes.

Well, time and tears went by and I collected dust.
For there were many things I didn't know.
When daddy went away, he said, try to be a man.
And someday you'll understand."[34]

Many daddies don't say much, letting their lives do the speaking by default. Then the kids are left to decipher the meaning. It is hard to counterfeit actions, but sometime it is harder to interpret them. Some things must be said. Use plain language to tell what motivated and informed your life's decisions and what lessons you have learned. Even if it is still a mystery to you, give it a shot. Move the ball down the field even if you can't get it into the end zone. Your kids will have a better chance at putting points on the board starting on the forty than just receiving the kickoff deep in the end zone. Get on with it now because "someday never comes."

Sons rely on their papas for important knowledge and papas are letting them down. Less due to lack of experience than a lack of willingness to think about it and speak, less often cowardice than apathy, and less often apathy than procrastination. Sons, for their part, are often not intentional about pursuing their fathers, not knowing what they're missing. Both assume someday they will get around to it or someday life will deliver the perfect opportunity and perfect information. You better get with it now if you want someday to ever come.

"I am here to tell you now,
Each and every mother's son,
That you better learned fast,
You better learn it young,
'Cause someday never comes."

Credence's message then and now is, "Figure it out and pass it on." Whether the bell has rung or not, get on with it. It's too important to ignore. Sons, chase down your fathers and, fathers, pass on the baton. Sons desperately need to know what fathers have to say. The baton needs to be passed and sons need to see how it is done. Their turn is next.

Moms and daughters are probably better at this; they have more words. I'll bet there are some things the XX chromosome set need to work too, but it is safer for me to not opine on that.

Advice for Passing the Baton

- Translate your failures into warnings, your successes in to significance, and launch all those you care about into their future off your shoulders.
- The baton passes need to be planned in the backstretch, then executed with words in the far corner, and reinforced with your life throughout.
- The homestretch should be left entirely for applause.
- It's not about duty, it's about opportunity. It is not about strapping another "to do" list on your already weary back, but an opportunity to prepare a final gift of words for those who desperately need to hear them.
- Your story is not your own. It is meant to be shared for good.
- Use plain language to tell what motivated and informed your life's decisions and what lessons you have learned.
- Offer your story as a gift.

The Home Stretch

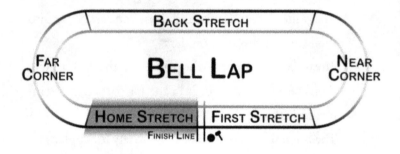

When your last remission comes to an end and you accept that there is no more treatment worth taking, you're on the homestretch. There is little telling how long it will last. It could be weeks, but if you have been bold enough to not take the worthless stuff it may be months, unlikely days or years. You don't have to figure it all out; you just have to admit that you can't.

Conclusion

The Home Stretch

> *"When it comes your time to die, be not like the folks whose hearts are filled with the fear of death so that when their time comes they weep and pray for a little more time to live their life over again in a different way. Sing your death song and live your life like a hero going home."* (Tacumseh, a Shawnee Chieftain in *Legends of the Fall*)

When that dreaded day of abandoning treatment arrived for Tom and he had recovered from the immediate shock of its arrival, he felt a sweet release. The burden to perform had vanished; there was nothing more *he* could do to lengthen his life, but much *he* could do to increase its value. There will be much you can still do to make your life count when/if that day arrives, too.

In a stadium, the homestretch is always right in front of the bleachers where everyone stands cheering as exhausted runners give it their all. The bell lap's homestretch is different. The fans are not expecting to watch a performance, they're expecting to share in an experience, and they have come with eyes and hearts of grace.

The work of the first stretch and the near corner are long past. The legal and financial issues long since resolved (or should be!) Anger, denial, depression, and bargaining have long ago been hurtled or abandoned. The charades of your life have hopefully been discovered through backstretch reflections. Wounds have been uncovered, healing has begun, strained relationships are mending, and new hopes for the next generation transmitted. The far corner has been a rewarding time of first recognizing the blessings of your own life and then taking the revealed wisdom and passing it on. The home stretch has arrived, but the exhausted deathbed times are still ahead.

Now you will have more time, albeit less energy, to ensure those batons have been safely transferred and none are lying dropped on the track. If they are, pick them up and pass them again with a smile. If humility was lost during the halcyon days of your successes, its return can warm and open the hearts of your audience. Now, at last, the homestretch is an unburdened time to be shared in lavish celebration. All those who have come to see life as a gift cannot be diminished now by suffering.

It is a time for reminiscing, valuing, validating, laughing and cheering, all those things that take place at the best memorial services: speeches, stories, testimonials, applause, clapping and high fives, all awash in tears and hugs. If you have planned your run well, escaped the fear driven invitation to give one last chemotherapy regimen a try (which is invariably worthless), then you will get to be present and soak it all in. Bask in the accolades and smiles, suffocate wonderfully in the hugs, share the tears of friendships long cherished, drink to the toasts, and fall to sleep once again in the arms of the one you love.

If you are the one coming down the home stretch, you can't orchestrate all of this, but you must tell those who can when you are ready to get started. You must have run the rest of the lap by now and run it well enough to be really ready. Hopefully they have run at your side and are ready, too. If you or they are still stuck in anger and denial or still harboring unresolved bitterness and regret, you will never be ready to celebrate. You will simply miss out and lose out on the celebration of your life. Then it will only take place after you're gone and in some sterile, after-the-fact memorial service and newspaper obituary.

The sooner you overcome the challenges of the earlier four segments of the race, the sooner you will be ready to get on with the celebrations and as many as possible. They can be rich and wonderful even if there is only an audience of one, but even more fun if there are many.

Ken did it well. Many marveled at just how well he did do it, and wondered just how he could. The sounding of his bell had been as strident and startling as it could be for anyone. One day he was a completely well man of fifty-five, actively engaged in life, family, and work. The next, he was learning he had a Stage 4 high-grade lymphoma threatening his life in short order. He marshaled the stamina to endure surgery and aggressive chemotherapy, chasing a cure, and was rapidly rewarded with a complete remission, but it didn't last long.

Fortunately, he had attended to the business of the first stretch immediately and then fought his way around the first corner clearing every hurdle. Then he had settled into a comfortable stride in the backstretch, made easier because he had already done a lot of the healing and contemplative work in his life before cancer showed up.

Most people learn to pull ahead of the Dragon in the backstretch and it doesn't really mind as long as it can reach out and scorch them with a little fire breath and fear now and then to show them it is still in control. Ken left it in the dust and wasted no energy dealing with it, so he was able to run free, fast, and unafraid. The uncertainties of remission somehow didn't seem to bother him. He slept well and kept smiling. He devoted his considerable stamina to family and even took on new projects at work and in the community.

Meanwhile, the Dragon didn't quit the race. It knew that most folks slow down in the far corner and become vulnerable again to attack. So, it just hung back waiting to sprint to catch Ken deep in the far corner. When Ken relapsed for the second time, he was still in pretty good health. There were some third line drugs (not good enough to use initially or with the first relapse) and even some new research drugs we could try, but it was clear there was no treatment with any chance of cure or meaningful remission (i.e. a feel good time of months or years).

The Dragon was right there oozing with charm and deceit and whispering, "Don't believe the doctor; it couldn't possibly be that bad; you feel too good; of course the medicine will work; you deserve for it to work; you are such a good person and have done so many good things and even prayed; show them you have grit; God is powerful and miracles still happen; sign up for more chemo and delicious hope, then claim your miracle."

Ken blew off the dragon and accepted the bad news with equanimity. He told me that to take more treatment would most likely mean the remainder of his life would be spent in doctors' offices and occupied by receiving drugs, taking tests, and recovering from side effects. He had known this time would arrive someday and had been preparing for the decisions he would need to make when it did. He had pondered and prayed about them and was ready to decide the moment they came.

He simply decided to forgo any more treatment and to focus on running the home stretch with all the passion he could muster. He started the celebrations himself. He gathered together groups of people that he had known or worked with for one last time, so he could tell them how much he had enjoyed them and how much he valued their friendship. He always made it clear he was still living even while dying. The celebrations were part of life, not a rolling memorial service. Without any prompting, friends reciprocated and created more events. The reminiscing was rich, the hugs heartfelt, and the laughter uplifting.

Then when he lived longer than anyone expected, there were more celebrations, more times of sharing, more laughter, and more trips. As Ken got more tired, others arranged the gatherings. Different groups, different places, different interests, but one common friendship, one universal bond of having lived life together, lives full of challenges, some disappointments, some failures, some successes, but all with a rich shared humanity.

Ken was not a powerful man, nor a rich man, nor a celebrity, but a family man, a lover, and a servant. He ran well and humbly. He got more time than anyone expected and finished strong leaving an indelible mark on everyone who knew him. He felt blessed to have no chemotherapy toxicity and enough energy to run the homestretch his way.

His final days were spent at home drifting in and out of a natural sleep caressed by a haze of morphine. Family would come and go. Grandchildren would climb all over him and play with blocks on his bed as he snoozed. They were too young to speak and the adults didn't need to. All the words had been said and there was no need for any more. Touch could say it all and could affirm the loving connections that his life had created, and a bell lap, well run, had cemented.

Ken was in a hospital bed by the living room picture window facing the sunrise when he breathed his last. Everyone wasn't present, but in a way everyone was, as the connections they shared with Ken and reaffirmed down the home stretch transcend time and space.

Ken was one of the Windrunners and he showed the world how to make a Bell Lap into a Victory Lap!

You too can make your bell lap a victory lap. For how the Windrunners were able to outrun and evade then defeat the Dragon see, CANCER'S WINDRUNNERS.

Appendix 1

A Word to Family, Caregivers, and Pacesetters

Caring for the dying is the truest form of love.

–Mother Teresa

Precious and Vital

Thank God for the support team and the caregivers. No one can run a bell lap without you. They can crawl maybe, but not run. You are the true friends. You are ever so precious. You are the encouragers, the listeners, the pacesetters, the nurses, medics, coaches, and counselors. You offer the certainty that there will be a witness to their lives and that they are valued.

You will find yourselves collectively on the track, running the lap right alongside your patient. You have got to keep up or lead. If you fall behind, you'll slow the runner down. So, you must treat this as if it were your own bell lap. You'll be in better shape if and when your own turn comes if you have run this practice lap and until then, the rest of your life will be richer for it.

Even though you are not the patient, you may go through some or all of Dr. Kubler-Ross' stages of reaction to terminal illness with them or on your own: denial and isolation, anger, bargaining, and depression before reaching the acceptance that allows you to run free. Be alert to what each stage might look like; be intentional in dealing with each one so that you can help your patient do the same. Every stage is disconcerting, but living through them is easier with a companion. Be that companion, but don't be mistaken into thinking that's all you are. If you can really imagine yourself facing your own death, you may be able to take your own spiritual journey to new depths and heights, and become more than a caregiver—maybe a virtual runner, maybe a pacesetter.

Know that one person cannot do it all. An effective caregiver must marshal a team early and keep every member involved right from the beginning, even if only in small ways. It is far better to have a few of your teammates complaining about riding the bench on the sidelines early in the game than to be shorthanded going into the fourth quarter.

One thing that is often overlooked, but that you can and should do early on is to construct a care plan that will enable everyone to stay the course. Compassion fatigue is very real and affects every caregiver sooner or later. It is hard to see it coming. It grows insidiously and chips away at your resolve to do what you have intended. The longer the course, the rougher it gets, the more you are needed, the more likely that burnout will take its toll. The antidote to this is to design your care plan to specifically provide for relief for yourself by planning and requiring rest, diversion, and refreshment. Above all, don't feel guilty about providing for your own as well as other caregivers' needs. This is essential if you are to be effective and persevere.

Caregivers are no better prepared for their role than the sick are prepared for theirs. The challenge for both is to keep the care-giving and the illness in their proper places. This is hardest when your efforts go unnoticed, unvalidated, and unrelieved. Your team has to do this for each other.

You must be intentional about taking care of yourself for the patient's sake. Take timeouts, run, ride, read, walk, and nap. Do all the things that feed your own soul and fill your love tank so you can be and do your best. Pace yourself by sharing the load with other team members. It will be richer for everyone. Every race has a home stretch and every care-giving team needs to be fit and prepared for it; there are always unforeseeable and exhausting new challenges.

Don't be surprised or feel guilty if the person you are caring for turns the tables and winds up caring for you. Let it be. It may be their way of thanking you or redressing past disharmonies when words seem too difficult.

Go with Them

When cast in a patient role, we are all somewhat discombobulated. Our normal faculties become compromised in unpredictable ways. The foreign medical environment is disconcerting to everyone, often compelling us to surrender much of our time and autonomy. This is when an attentive caregiver/team member who goes along to appointments can run interference by reporting symptoms, representing needs, taking notes, gathering information, keeping the calendar, managing the schedule, and listening, listening, listening. Later, they can be an invaluable source of facts and perspective for both the patient and family.

I encourage patients and caregivers to be assertive with the medical community. Ask lots of hard questions. Press through for the hard answers. Press past the *change-of-subject-sidesteps* some physicians use when confronted with hard issues. Press until you get an answer, or an "I don't know." Then ask, "When will we know?" and "Will we ever know?" or "Who else should I ask?" Take a tape recorder with you and just turn it on at the beginning of the visit. Many patients do this because the doctor's office is often a stress induced brain-dead zone. *Working memory* is what we use to manipulate new information so it can be integrated with remote memory. The average individual can only juggle six to ten new bits of information before adding another bit will cause others to drop off. In my experience, this number decreases with stress, foreignness of the information, patient age, and pain medications.

As cancer information is all new, it will be displaced rapidly. Emotionally charged information displaces what is already on the bench even faster. If data is not understood, categorized and integrated, it is not transformed into long-term memory. Instead, it is lost. When needed for decision making twelve to fifteen bits later, patients are out of luck. Caregivers can collect their own ten bits and hang on to them better when they are less emotionally involved, but a tape recorder gets it all.

The recorder can be particularly valuable to playback for absent family members who may have a role in decision-making or simply need to be accurately informed. When I have spoken to a family about what they have been told by the patient regarding our office visit, I have been astonished at how little of what I have said made it home accurately or at all.

This can be critical when it applies to how to take medications. A recording can supplement a written record. It is a good idea to keep a small ring binder that can travel to each appointment with the patient and be passed from teammate to teammate to serially record specific physician instructions. If the caregiver takes the notes, it lets the patient focus on what the doctor saying. The binder can also be used at home as a log for recording side effects and symptoms, questions for the next visit, the use of pain medications, and their efficacy over time. All of these are often forgotten by the time the next physician's appointment rolls around.

It's Hard to Run Weighed Down

Know your patient's concerns and address them. Two-thirds of patients are weighed down and concerned about being a burden to others. In fact, it is their number one concern, followed closely by a fear of being separated from loved ones and next by a concern for how their loved ones will manage after their death, feelings of worthlessness, and lack of purpose. Whenever you can provide reassurance, reaffirm their value, help them discover purpose, it will chase the clouds away, but those clouds often return, so make you reassurance a routine. It is such an easy way to love on them and just what they need.

To the extent patients have allowed their work, appearance, skills, avocations or their relationships define them, they are vulnerable to the whims of an illness that can so easily alter all of those. Anyone who has ever dealt with self-doubt, low self-esteem, self-rejection or depression is likely to have illness re-create the darkness of those feelings. You can be an empathetic witness to their adversities and validate their feelings, and at the same time question the accuracy of their conclusions. You can address each one head on and will need to do it repeatedly. You can speak the truth of their goodness and their belovedness, their value to you, family, and friends and most of all by their God. If faith is your fortress, you can remind them that they are God's chosen precious creation and encourage them on their spiritual journey where they can discover that truth for themselves. When appropriate, recruit a priest, a Stephen Minister or a trained counselor to help.

When there is grief, let them lead in expressing it. Be cautious in expressing your own grief around them as you don't want to quash whatever hope and hunger they still have for living by making them feel already dead.

Read this book with the others on your team about the issues patients encounter coming off the starting line and through the near corner, so you all can help your patient deal with feelings of denial, fear, and anger by asking questions as well as being a sounding board. Some patients disappear into themselves and a black hole of sour feelings. They need to be drawn out to understand and process all they are feeling. Help them put a face on their fears (faces of the dragon) to give them a target to deal with. Keep your fears to yourself, they don't need them.

Communications with Family, Friends, and the Team

Start a blog or register on Caring Bridge, a website for connecting people when someone who is ill, and make posts regularly. It gives your patient a voice when they are too tired to keep up with phone calls and visits, and serves to keep everyone up-to-date including those close family members who may be called on to participate in care or decisions. It enables everyone to be processing the realities as they emerge and provides a conduit for them to express their concern and affection which a patient can choose to receive on their own schedule.

When cancer strikes someone, it strikes a whole family. The dynamics will change. It is like one person in a small lifeboat has shifted positions and everyone else has to be paying attention to move around and change roles/positions to keep the boat from capsizing. It all needs to be done while honoring their needs without tripping over pity, neither disenfranchising the one who is sick nor turning them into a control monger. Assist them in retaining as much of their identity as possible, until they can redefine and reinvent themselves, separate and distinct from their disease.

Be aware that there are a lot of commonly accepted roles that patients find themselves forced into: the brave, the cheerful, the godly, the good patient, the non-complainer, the fighter— particularly within their family. There is nothing wrong with any of these roles unless they are a role assigned by others or a smokescreen to hide fear and insecurity.

Most everyone can benefit from a confidant outside the family who can be a safe place where real feelings can come out in the open, free from the interpersonal spousal or sibling politics. If you can be that person, just listen. It is probably wise to hold off on giving guidance until asked. Just be present and tactful.

Yesterday, a friend recounted how he had struggled for forty-eight hours trying to figure out what to say to someone with newly diagnosed cancer and what advice he might give. Without ever figuring that out, he just called his friend and discovered how grateful his buddy was just to be called and what that alone meant. It was much easier than he expected. The patient didn't want advice; he just wanted caring connection. Frankly, the last thing a patient wants or needs is unsolicited advice, especially since they will receive plenty of it anyway during the course of their treatment.

Be sensitive to your patient's mood and tactful in how you phrase questions. There is a difference between asking the usual, "How are you feeling?" and "Do you want me to ask how you are feeling?" The first is more intrusive and demanding while the second is gentler and allows the person to say no on the days he/she is feeling well and doesn't want to focus on being the sick person or is doing badly and doesn't want to be reminded of it or has already answered that question too many times. Whenever possible, avoid asking if there are things you can do, just do them, thereby avoiding reminding people of their dependence. [35]

When the time is right, there are three questions that need to be asked repeatedly and pondered delicately, ones that physicians seldom ask, which, when answered, can dramatically affect an individual's quality of life and guide your care.

What are you afraid of?
What are your goals this week and this year?
What outcome for you would not be acceptable?[36]

Use Books to Connect and Fill the Void

Read out loud just as you did to children; it's a comforting connection. Read books to each other or independently then discuss them. Beyond the sheer entertainment value, books can shift the focus of one's mind away from self and cancer. They can be counted on to be there when the time is right and a delicious escape without the inconvenience of a TV schedule or the strife it so often depicts.

The subject matter can give two people a chance to talk about all kinds of things, even anxious subjects that are hard to bring up. A couple to consider in that vein that are entertaining as well as provocative are the classic, *Crossing to Safety* by Wallace Stegnar, which is about a the lifelong relationship between two couples, and *Deadline* by Randy Alcorn, a murder mystery with spiritual insights.

Make Plans, Have Fun, and be Flexible

Reminiscing is always good. Visit places in the car and in pictures taking time to relive the fun associations that go with each.

Before leaving for the day, make plans for where you will travel on your next visit. Illness and age can steal dreams, so every time you can set out a plan for tomorrow or next week, it helps fill the void and lets them enjoy the anticipation.

Moods are contagious so be sure yours is uplifting, and corral others who can do the same. Protect patients from those whose attempts at compassion become an opportunity to unload their own fears and anxieties. Be assertive and change the subject and the friend. Those who are confused about their own life's journey need more care than they can give, but they can still help. Ask them to meet physical needs like meal preparation, chores, bill paying, etc., but perhaps it is best to avoid the one-on-one times where they can be more of a burden.

Steer conversations to fun and funny past events. Plan movie times out or rent fun ones with happy endings. These are particularly important when folks are on pain medications which compromise short term memory. Movies and novels with many characters or complex plots can be difficult and distressing. It is hard to enjoy reading a story when you can't remember what you read on the last page. Coffee table picture books, albums, and National Geographic can all overcome this problem, providing a whole experience on one page. Likewise, travel log videos like Planet Earth or documentaries can provide entertainment in the moment without having to recall all the key points of plot development in a typical movie.

In cataclysmic moments, no words are as eloquent as an embrace. Sadly, many families and especially dads can forget the relational vocabulary of touching and hugging that came so naturally when the kids were young. When moments are supercharged with emotion, even the words at one's command may just not be enough. Only a touch, an embrace or gazing deeply into another's eyes can connect souls and then words become unnecessary.

Look deeply, hold your gaze, and hug those you love often. Hold hands, and when you can, get everyone's hand in the pile like the beginning of a basketball game or in a circle, just connect! It may take practice, but you will never regret it and it shows the kids how it's done. If you don't, the risk is that vital feelings may never find expression. It is a time when loneliness and separation can grow. Don't let a chance for affirmation or healing pass you by. Reach out. Overcome it. It just takes a hand!

It's not just for family. I learned that subliminally as a child watching my physician father comfort his patients on house calls and hospital rounds. Since then, I have held more hands and hugged more patients than I can count. It has meant as much to me as I suspect it did to them. Sometimes, mine were the only hands they held and hugs they got. Sometimes, touch did all the talking. Never pass up a chance; most everyone is hungry for what touch brings.

Sometimes, during family visits the silence in a patient's room is deafening. There is so much to say, but so few with courage to speak. They just don't know what to say. Start by telling stories and reminiscing, and then retell the good ones over and over again. If the patient is either elderly or on pain medications, the odds are they will remember the event of years past, but will have forgotten what you just talked about it yesterday and will get to enjoy it all over again.

Sometimes, walking into a family conference one is greeted by the stench of rotting family relationships. Cancer is a great revealer, not the creator of family tensions. It exposes fraudulent love, codependence, and other addictions. Cancer can easily defeat anyone's self-centered agenda and out comes the ugliness. It is unlikely that the hardhearted and blind are going to soften and regain their sight in these situations, so the best one can do is damage control by limiting exposure.

Other times, one family member can initiate healing for another. In one such moment, Alice helped her sister experience their father's love, acceptance, and forgiveness by saying, "Dad, Betsy has always felt she failed you by marrying Joe against your wishes. Is there anything you can say to her about that?" The marriage had not just ended, but ended disastrously as predicted. The girls' father, a man of stature and power, now mellowed by the years and illness, turned to Betsy and reaching out a hand said, "Ahh, you were young and didn't know what you were doing. It's okay, it happens." He couldn't quite add on the "I love you," but it was enough for Betsy. Years of self-recrimination melted away.

A bruised love mended, a burden lifted, and so few words needed. Healing happens in many ways. Team up and go after it.

Celebrate

Mistakenly, many of us create a fantasy of happiness dreaming about the future. When cancer threatens to take that away, feelings of emptiness and worthlessness are hard to avoid. Cancer cannot take away the wonderful experiences one has had even if there were not enough— the happiness, the goodness, or the lives touched, the relationships, the achievements, and the challenges surmounted. Nothing can remove these. They are worthy of celebration. These things did matter and they will always matter. They need to be rescued from the nearly forgotten past and celebrated. Done well and repeatedly, these celebrations can fill the void of the vanishing future. It takes committed family and caregivers to make these things happen over and over again. As intangible as reminiscences are, these celebrations are in themselves often the best real medicine. They're available every day, and each one will inspire another. Over time, they will validate who we were, who we still are, and who we will always be.

Disease may change what we can do, but it should not change who we are. Illness distracts us and many just walk away from themselves. Friends and family can prevent that from happening with frequent reminders. You can make the medicine last longer if you schedule events in the future and then relish both the anticipation before and the reminiscence after.

Another way to focus on your patient's worthiness is to help them discover the batons they have to pass and who they can pass them to. Then help create the situations where these baton passes can occur and celebrate each successful pass.

The Breaking Point Discussion

Family members can play a vital role by initiating breaking point conversations early. There comes a time to switch from fighting for more days to live to fighting for more comfort to live meaningfully. That is the point when patients break away from more cancer treatment, more tests, and more doctor visits to focus on the care of their heart, soul, friends, and family.

Before a patient gets to those heavy discussions, help them go over the *Gotta Do List*. Once those issues are dealt with, confront the unavoidable fact that a time will come when chemotherapy will no longer work or be worth taking. Start ferreting out just how one will know that time to break away has arrived. Will the breaking point be defined by how broken down and awful one feels, by how unlikely there will be benefit, by when the doctor throws in the towel, or by when they grab it and leave the ring?

I would encourage the latter, but if it is to be the former, one must define how much someone is willing to go through to sustain their illusion of living, and what level of being alive is worth fighting for. Is sleeping and watching TV enough? Is hand holding and listening to a voice enough for you or for them? Or is being out of bed and engaged in activities essential? There may come a time when some will consider oxygen at home, or a feeding tube or another surgery. Other illness may intervene such as pneumonia, dehydration or stroke, raising the question of another possible admission to the hospital. Patients are often too tired and beaten down by their disease to anticipate upcoming questions or deal with them when they arrive. However, the decisions will need to be made and will be made better if made proactively.

A wise caregiver can initiate the *what-if* conversations and coax out tentative decisions early including a negotiated consensus with the family if necessary. Such discussions compel all family members to become informed and to work through the issues prospectively, so that everyone can hopefully end up on the same page and avoid a calamity of confusion and conflicting wills at critical moments.

Stepping over the breaking point is a courageous and victorious step. A huge weight comes off of the shoulders of everyone who takes that step. If family and friends all take that step together with the patient, then another weight is lifted, and they can all run down the home stretch together. Reread the Home Stretch chapter and figure out how you can facilitate or participate in a celebration of a life all down the home stretch.

Palliative Care and Hospice

Since caring for the dying moved out of the home into the hospital in the mid-1900s, there's a whole generation without personal experience in rendering such care at home. It is not technologically difficult, but it can be more physically exhausting than one might imagine or than it need be. With the advent of hospice care in the late '70s and its growing availability today, care at home for the dying is changing. It is best started early than too late.

It is not one size fits all. Once started, the frequency and intensity of care can be adjusted. Often, there are palliative care programs that can be initiated even while active anticancer therapy is ongoing. With their help and advice, caregivers can optimize this time for everyone even if it lasts weeks or months. It can be a special, tender, and meaningful time rather than an exhausting desperate one.

For those who have an incurable disease, you cannot have your initial consultation with these services too early. Sadly, many wait for a referral from their oncologist, many of whom have difficulty talking about end-of-life issues and routinely overestimate patient life spans. Referral to palliative or hospice care by oncologists is often made only when no other treatment option of any kind remains. Patients are often unable to let go of even mediocre treatment options until they understand there is another option: hospice.

In a study at Harvard, researcher, Nicholas Cristakis, interviewed doctors caring for some 500 terminally ill patients to estimate how long they thought their patients would survive. Sixty-three percent of the physicians grossly overestimated the survival time and were often off by several hundred percent.[37] More than 40 percent of oncologists even reported offering treatments that they believed were unlikely to work. This is partly because it is painful and time-consuming for doctors to talk about death issues and partly because they don't want to trample upon a patient's expectations (which the doctors themselves may have falsely created).

Patients are often loath to consult hospice on their own, as if doing so would hasten their death. Sometimes, they fear they will not receive enough medical care once hospice is involved. Both ideas are wrong.

The only randomized trial to examine standard cancer care, with and without hospice support, showed no significant difference in survival rates, but did show significant improvements in quality of life when cancer care and hospice care were combined.

"Preliminary analysis revealed a 27 percent cost reduction in the combined-care group, which received less chemotherapy and diagnostic testing by choice and required fewer hospitalizations"[38] (*New England Journal of Medicine*). This fits with the national statistics that 25 percent of all Medicare spending is for the 5 percent of patients who are in their final year of life, and most of that money goes for care in the last couple of months which, by definition, is of little apparent benefit or the patient wouldn't have died.

The truth is that for most cancers, chemotherapy doesn't do much if any good after someone relapses the third time, and has only marginal benefit after the second relapse. It sidetracks priorities, wastes people's precious time, and depletes everyone's health care dollars. Insist the physician prove to you what good will come from more chemo after a third relapse before you take it. There are exceptions to this rule, most notably breast cancer and lymphomas, but they are few. So, put your physician to the test before you support your patient's signing up for one.

Both palliative care programs and hospice offer compassionate counseling regarding what to expect in the late stages of illness. They are skilled to palliate symptoms and improve quality of life. Having an initial consultation does not mean signing up for biweekly visits, but starts an educational process and gets one registered in the system so that it will be available when needed.

Studies have demonstrated that patients with advanced cancer who have had candid end-of-life discussions with their physicians regarding their expected survival and the effectiveness of additional treatment often opted for less aggressive medical care.

When more aggressive care was chosen, it was associated with worse quality of life for patients and more depression among caregivers, whereas longer hospice involvement was related to better quality of life for patients as well as for caregivers.[39] Positive associations were found between end of life discussions, patient mental health, medical care near death, and caregiver bereavement adjustment. Our technology can sustain our organs until we are well past the point of awareness and coherence, even beyond suffering, but leave our families trapped in it! May we all have caregivers brave enough to make the tough decisions and spare us from such technology.

Many people believe that hospice care hastens death because its patients forgo hospital care. However, studies suggest otherwise. No difference in survival times is found in comparing hospice patients and non-hospice patients with breast, prostate, and colon cancer. Curiously, hospice care was associated with prolonged survival in pancreatic and lung cancer (probably because they avoided worthless third or fourth line chemo) as well as congestive heart failure. Patients gained an average of three weeks, six weeks, and three months respectively. It seems you live longer, only when you stop trying to live longer. I have observed this repeatedly.

The most common final pathway toward death for cancer patients is liver failure due to cancer destroying liver function. As we normally have far more liver function available than we actually use regularly, a lot can be destroyed by a growing cancer before we get many symptoms. But there is a threshold amount of vital liver function that is absolutely necessary and when it is breached, death can come surprisingly fast, catching many off guard.

A very gradual decline can become precipitous. The only hint of change being an enlarging liver with declining function as detected by rising liver enzymes in the blood. Family may notice increased fatigue and loss of appetite. Jaundice (yellowing of the eye whites) may appear, but is a late and unreliable sign.

I caution patients and families that when cancer is growing in the liver to a significant degree, it is like ice-skating on a frozen pond as spring arrives. Day after day a skater can race and dance on the ice even while it is melting. Then after one warmer day, the ice melts one more vital millimeter, i.e. the liver function declines one more iota, and the skater crashes through and is all wet, and the cancer patient declines rapidly to death's doorstep. Family members can be left holding their plane tickets 1,000 miles away wondering what has happened. Don't wait that long. Better they come early and get some quality time, than miss out altogether.

While the rapidity with which it happens is often dramatic, the associated symptoms seldom are. Profound fatigue sends the afflicted to bed and the appetite disappears. If shortness of breath or pain have been problems, they may accelerate toward the end, but both can be controlled by alert hospice nurses and the generous use of morphine and other medications. If for some reason you feel your patient is not getting the care necessary, be in direct contact with the physician; return to standard care and a hospital is always an option.

May your "caring for the dying be your truest form of love" and may your hearts swell with the silent gratitude of those who could give no more and deserve no less.

Cancer's
WindRunners

Spirit Powered
Hope Energized
The Dragon Vanquished

Robert F Lane, M.D.

XULON PRESS

PREFACE
CANCER'S WINDRUNNERS

Cancer can be **defeated every time**, so **why** is it so terrifying for everyone?

It is because it attacks **the life you live**
    not just the body you live in.
It is because it attacks the life you live
    more than the body you live in.
It is because it affects most of the life you live **most of the time**
    while it attacks some of the body some of the time.

It's not just about biology, it's about spirituality.
It's not about what is out of your control,
It's about what is in the center of your control!

Let the Windrunners show you how.

I was jogging along Hood Canal on a hot August afternoon with a salt breeze in my face and the familiar scent of crushed madrone leaves underfoot. However, I was not feeling the familiar exhilaration of running: time alone, no phone, no schedule, no pain, just freedom, beauty, and a chance just to think. I had spent years focused on becoming a physician and NOW Three years out of training I was doing research, practicing hometown oncology, earning a living, but I was also totally bedraggled and beat up. Not burned out from working hours too long and too intense, but burned up because too many people were dying on my shift. No more than other oncologists, but still just too many. Cancer was winning JUST too often.

These were not just my patients; these were my friends. I knew their families and their dreams, and they knew mine. Together we had beaten back their disease, often several times; we had both celebrated and cried. No matter how many triumphs, there were just too many tears and too many deaths.

In training I had rotated from service to service, seldom seeing the same patient for more than a few months. Real medical practice was different because I was with the same patients for the long haul. There were lots of cures and remissions, but too often, the long haul became the final haul. That hurt... too much and felt like failure... too often.

For the first time while running along by the water, indecision struck. Maybe this is not what I am cut out for? Maybe I should do something different? What a miserable thought!

Being a man of some spiritual knowledge and a sometimes faith, I started to pray; something I had little experience with except in the foxholes of my life. I poured out my confusion and despondency to my sometimes God. Without remembering just what I said, I do recall with crystal clarity what He said, especially because I don't think I had ever heard Him say anything before.

"I have got you exactly where I want you!"

Startled and confused thoughts tumbled out. "Whoa! Where did that come from? Could that be God? What a presumptuous idea! Does God really speak out loud? And to guys like me?"

I concluded it just might be. A look around quickly revealed I was all alone and it sure wasn't me. At first I thought "that's cool," but then other thoughts flooded in. "What a bad idea. I don't like it and what does it mean?"

That is when I heard, **"It's not if they die; it is what happens before they die that matters!"**

So I told him. It seemed to mean that everyone is going to die sooner or later and the timing was up to Him. Yet, there also appeared to be something terribly important was supposed to happen first which was up to us. Apparently, my role could and should be more than I imagined, more than I had been taught. They were coming to me for treatment. Yet, at a more visceral level, they were coming for hope, and there was so much more to hope than just the medicine I was offering. I wasn't sure what it was and spent a few years sorting it out, but in that moment my focus shifted and expanded. I felt a sense of commission. Despondency seemed to disappear, and in its place came a new sense of purpose and possibility.

Thirty years later, and six months before my scheduled retirement, someone I had been getting to know awakened me at 3:00 A.M. with a compulsion, **"It is time to write what I have been teaching you."** Again, I thought it must be God because such an audacious idea was the furthest thing from my mind.

It happened twice before I finally got up and started to write. I knew it wasn't my voice or my idea because I had done everything in my science-focused education to avoid writing. This book is a testimony to the One who could distract me from all my beloved outdoor pursuits and plant me in front of a keyboard to write it.

The years and my patients have been hands-on teachers and their lessons have been profound. There was a group of patients beset by a tragic diagnosis whose lives refused to become tragic. It was not because of what I did or what they did. Yet, invariably, they were victorious. I was astonished. Sometimes, they me told what they learned on their journeys; other times I learned from just watching them. Still other times, I learned in the dark and scary hours of my own journey.

Windrunners

Something unique was going on with those patients. They were doing better than the rest and the Dragon was nowhere to be seen. You met the Dragon in the last book, *Cancer's Bell Lap and The Dragon Behind The Door,* and learned how it disabled so many people in both their lives and their fight against cancer.

It was a patient and a friend, Sue, who so eloquently described how the Dragon haunted her, and how she dealt with it. Since then, countless patients and even some non-patients have identified with Sue's experience with that metaphorical Dragon.

"It would show up at the darnedest times, sometimes in the middle of the night and other times just as contentment or happiness was about to break out. There it was. Always a spoiler," she said.

They all described it as jeering voices in their heads of personal frailty or inadequacy, voices of the media fostering desire and discontent, and the voices of evil itself always whispering:

"You're going to miss out."

"Time is going to run out."

"What if?"

"Not enough."

"What if?"

And still more, "What if?"

No one could kill this Dragon, outrun it, hide from it, or cover it up with all kinds of beautiful stuff. Some were able to defeat it and run Bell Laps unhindered by it. What a mystery it all seemed. I had caught a glimpse of something true and have been in search of the fullness of that truth ever since. It wasn't their fitness, nor their ethnicity, nor the type or stage of their cancer. It was not their gender, age, education, or religion, but it was real, and it brought them peace and comfort amid turmoil and terror. Everyone at the cancer center could feel it and see it, but not pinpoint exactly what it was at first. Yet it set these patients apart. Despite the challenges of a Bell Lap, they ran like the wind inviting me to think of them as, "The Windrunners." (Yes, I have coined the word for this book and in honor of those remarkable people.)

None of us grow into spiritual maturity by choice. We're usually dragged there by suffering or enticed there by mystery. Most of us are spiritually lazy, willing to stay on the same path we're already on even if it is going nowhere. To find a new path takes motivation and daring. Windrunners had both, and it led to an unexpected adventure.

Often, it wasn't until the bell rang that anyone could sense the difference; most everyone smiles in happy-snappy land. The Windrunners would generally separate from the pack right off the starting line, but not all of them. Some did not distinguish themselves until later. Something would change. They would move to the outside lane away from the Dragon, start pulling ahead of the pack in the backstretch, then fly round the far corner to join up with the rest of the Windrunners as they accelerated through the far corner and down the homestretch. Some are still running!

The Expanding Specter of Cancer

There are more people being cured of cancer today than thirty years ago, but that is largely due to earlier diagnosis of localized disease for which surgery and other treatments are more likely curative. The cure rate for advanced stage disease hasn't changed much while our ability to keep patients in remission longer has improved. The number of people living under the apprehension of relapse and eventual death, both those hopefully cured and those unlikely ever cured, has grown enormously and without knowing it become Dragon fodder!

They all live on the outskirts of hope; ever feeling and fearing that there is a Dragon behind the door. For some, the Dragon is very big and others not so much. Some deal with it every day, others not so often. *They all know it is there.* It taints the lives of all but a few while manipulating decisions of most and stealing joy from all.

The Dragon is a problem bigger than most cancers and produces an *illness* of social, emotional, interpersonal, and spiritual chaos. It strikes at every cancer patient's heart, to wear away many a desire, erode many a dream, and even corrupt many a thought.

Yet, some people can escape the hopelessness and deception. They not only defeat the Dragon, but smother it with irrelevancy by reframing the "what if?" question. They are the Windrunners.

This book is about them, the exceptions to the norm, the ones who ran faster, further, with more grace, and often longer.

(Real life invariably brings some suffering which is curiously a prerequisite for engaging this book. If you are as yet unscathed, you may be too young to understand that. But cancer will change everything. If still unscathed, I would wait a few months to begin the book.)

Who are they?
What makes their lives different?
What enables them to run their laps with such peace and purpose and even joy?
How is it they could finish so strong despite such a weakening and discouraging disease?
What does it take to be one of them?

They are the people I have known, loved, and cared for who have run (or still are running) what might be their last lap and doing it really well! None seemed to know how long it would last. None had ever run it before or knew what to expect. None knew what pains and fears would lie ahead. None knew what resources they would have or what others would bring. None of them knew who would be with them and who wouldn't or how the disease would end. Yet they knew something and had something that enabled them to run like the wind anyway. Somehow, they seemed to know already that the planned obsolescence of our bodies, though it wears them out or breaks them down, is meant to transform us. They had already willingly begun that process.

How do they do it?
Does it matter?
Can anyone do what they did?

Their stories will tell you that it does matter immensely and that you can do it, too. It can be easy, but it is seldom obvious. It has to do with spirituality, but not in a way you might think, and not in a way that was obvious to me. I was missing something. I didn't understand what it was until a totally unrelated, serendipitous event occurred and God took advantage of it to instruct me. It involved something golden brown covered with fur, eight feet tall with a long nose, teddy-bear ears, and a large hump between its shoulder blades. I was about to face the bear— literally and figuratively.

Guidelines for Reading this Book

What I am sharing with you is garnered from the lives of patients, the crucible in which they were purified and clarified. It is said that an author must have two essential qualities for sharing—expertise and experience. Thanks to my professional training and the wonderful patients I have learned from, I hope that the truths we experienced together can be the fodder for such a process in you.

However, the banquet of ideas is so rich they cannot likely be digested all at once. Consuming too much, too fast can lead to much of it running right through you not leaving behind much of nutritional value. It needs to be consumed and contemplated in a piecemeal fashion. So while the chapters are topical and may be contemplated all at once for a reflective study group, I suggest you go through this book the following way

1. You might want to skim over a whole chapter at first to get an overview of what's coming and then tackle one segment per day. If you need longer, take it. Don't rush. Journal and answer the questions.

2. So, most chapters are divided into five segments or approximately five days. Read each segment and then stop. At the end of each segment is a journal page. On that page write down any notes or important truths you want to remember, memorize, and/or reflect/meditate on. If you need more space than this book has allotted, then pick up a journal or empty notebook for gathering your thoughts, feelings, ideas, and truths.

3. Yes, you are also writing a book for yourself and perhaps a family member or friend. I encourage you to not only read this book yourself but to do it with another person. The two of you may wish to discuss, share, speak truth in love to one another, and even pray for or with each other. I remember the proverbial truth, "There is a friend who sticks closer than a brother."[1] Another one reads, "A sweet friendship refreshes the soul."[2]

---

[1] Proverbs 18:24b

[2] Proverbs 27:9 MSG

4. Take time to go through each chapter. Let its truths go deep into your soul so that like fine food that must marinate, your memory is saturated by what is real, lasting, and even eternal.

Our memory is like a workbench for our projects, but there is limited space and the bench get smaller with stress and age. Each time another project or idea gets added others get bumped off unless there has been time to integrate the new idea with the database you have already stored in long-term memory files. The bumped off ideas are lost and forgotten. If you mull over the new information, it is more likely to be remembered and integrated. The ideas, facts, truths, and wisdom build on one another like individual Lego pieces creating a weapon that will vanquish the Dragon and beat the cancer.

Chapter 1

Facing the Bear

I was all alone 3000 miles north of my Seattle home when it came rambling rudely into my life. It walked right out of the fever dreams of my childhood and out of the Yukon tundra and taught me something that not only my cancer patients, but God had been trying to teach me for years – something the Windrunners already knew. Naked from a plunge in an arctic stream before making the dinner campfire, I came face to face with an animal drawn to the smell of food and looking for dinner.

Any person has the capacity to learn profound things about oneself and God in a personal encounter with a horrible illness. I had watched them for years on the cancer wards, but I was a slow learner until I met Ursus Actos Horribilis. My bare nakedness was no match for his bear grizzliness. While I quickly lost my appetite, that grizzly did not.

Only when I rounded a scrub fir carrying my shirt and shorts did I see my gun and clothes lying across my pack at the feet of a very large bear squinting at me through beady black eyes. Its head swayed from right to left as it studied me. *I was without a weapon, a tree to climb, much of a plan or much of a faith. Odds of survival didn't look that good!*

I was caught completely by surprise, entirely vulnerable, defenseless, and alone; sort of the way cancer catches so many. I was cold with a clammy wetness and not just from the stream. My first inclination was to run, and so was my second.

Why is it that prayer, conversation with God, is mostly limited in our lives to moments of desperation instead of regular times of intimacy? In the crisis of facing a bear, somewhere down my to-do list came the thought, *Pray!* Meanwhile, the bear just stood there getting bigger by the second, kind of like the dawning specter of a just-diagnosed cancer. Sound familiar?

How very inconvenient it (any crisis) all was and how it spoiled all my plans. It interrupted what had been a marvelous day and promised to be a beautiful evening. Of course, I didn't think much about that; I was too busy just being scared. Much later, when the fear receded a little, I got really angry. That had more to do with getting my hands on a gun than being brave.

In the midst of that crisis, icy fear and intense anger took control. Thoughts of gratitude for still being alive were fleeting as fear and anger jockeyed for domination of my thoughts. How silly, ignoble, and arrogant of me to presume to be angry. The bear was only doing what bears do, following his nose towards food, and, in this case, me. ***Cancer just does what it does: grow continuously, invade, and then destroy other organs and lives.***

I am equally silly when I get upset with my body when it does what bodies do, i.e., break down. Dangerous and unpredictable *bears* will always appear in our lives, they just have different names. *The question isn't if crises (bears, dragons, diseases, etc.) will appear, but **when,** and **how** we will respond.*

That bear taught me something that many learn from cancer, and it will stand me in good stead whichever terror I face next.

Not many of us are as put together or secure as we think we are. Cancer can quickly reveal all the tiny cracks we are trying so hard to keep together. It can become an anvil on which so many lives are shattered, but that need not be the case. It does bring the key questions and obstacle of life into focus with great urgency for those paying attention.

In *The Bell Lap and The Dragon Behind the Door,* a cancer diagnosis became a metaphorical bell announcing possibly the last lap of a life. Not many recognize what that portends, neither the risks nor the opportunities, but those who do will address these key questions:

Who am I?

Why am I here?

What has God got to do with it?

How do I run a better and often longer Bell Lap?

DAY 1

A WINDRUNNER'S JOURNAL

I invite you to reread every sentence above which is bold and in italics. Write it down, in your own words if you wish, to remember it, reflect on it, discuss it, or even memorize it.

_____

_____

_____

_____

_____

_____

_____

_____

_____

_____

_____

_____

A Disease and an Illness

To begin to answer these questions, we need to understand cancer is both a disease and an illness. One affects your organs and the other your life. At first, you cannot detect either one until something vital stops working properly—either you hurt or your life hurts. *The disease comes from injured genes, toxins or a virus, while the illness comes from something I call the Dragon. The doctors battle the disease, but it is up to you to deal with the illness and the Dragon.*

God has given us life and the right to dispose of it as we choose. Cancer does not lessen the number of choices, but it increases the urgency to get the decisions right. *It will be your character choices about who you are and why you are here that will determine your destiny and your legacy as well as how happy you are along the way.* No cancer can steal your character from you and no friend or doctor can give it to you. You don't need to be talented or wealthy, smart or strong, but you do need a good model and mentor. Who will be yours be?

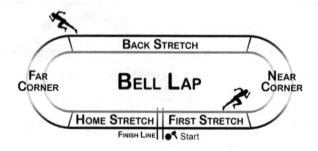

Both the disease and the illness, play out phase by phase over months and years. How does one grapple with two such foreign problems? The framework of running a race on an oval track and its Bell Lap helps us think sequentially about the phases of cancer and the strategies for living them. We dealt with a lot of the practical and medical aspects in the first book, but without including God in the equation. He doesn't want to foist Himself on anyone or be an obstacle for anyone in pursuit of practical knowledge, and I didn't want to do that for Him.

The cancer bell sounds to announce the beginning of what might be someone's final lap. Breathing hard down the first stretch, the cancer-scared runner reaches the near corner, endures treatment, and then rounds strongly into the remission backstretch. Relapse leads doggedly into the far corner which breaks breathlessly onto the home stretch ending graciously at the finish line.

The Dragon always appears on this lap and spews the very same life-altering, death-fearing illness into everyone's life sooner or later; if it is not already there. ***Cancer unmasks that Dragon by bringing it out in the open where we can see and experience the insidious drama of its actions.*** Everyone watching can recognize those who battle it victoriously and those who don't.

The Bell Lap and the Dragon behind the Door

My first book addressed the planning and preparation necessary in the first stretch after hearing the Bell. Then it introduces the Dragon in the near corner with its many voices as well as the various tools and tricks it employs to trip us up as we are trying to collect ourselves for the treatment and a different life ahead.

Those surviving that corner enter a backstretch of opportunity for spiritual reflection, discovery, and growth with an opportunity to optimize relationships and prepare to pass the batons of their life to the next generation. The far corner is a time for tough and critical decision making. While the homestretch is for celebration and anticipation for Windrunners, it brings fear and dread for everyone else.

Where Does God Fit In?

When the bell tolls, almost everyone at least fleetingly wonders, "What has God got to do with it?" Some set off on a spiritual journey which can make their Bell Lap as intensely a spiritual time as it is an intensely biologic, social, and economic time. Even those for whom everything spiritual smacks of hogwash start to wonder, "Does God have a role here? And, if so, how and what? Does it really make a difference?" Whether you are atheist, agnostic, Buddhist, Moslem, Hindu, or Christian, this time becomes one of dicey questioning, especially as you feel the heat of the Dragon's presence on the back of your neck and smell its breath.

Cancer can destroy a body, but it often destroys a life first. A battle must be engaged on both the biologic and the spiritual fronts, recognizing that with every victory on one front frees up energy and resources to commit to the other.

If my readers are anything like my patients, then I am speaking to a few who know God well, some who have just met Him, some who met Him long ago only to push Him onto a back shelf, some who were force-fed religion about Him only to walk away nauseated, and some who have never given anything spiritual much thought.

In the Cancer Center, I never knew to whom I was speaking, but I needed to speak to them all just as I want to with you right now. I have been in many of those same spiritual places myself and have wrestled with many of the same challenges. Please hang with me in those moments when I am writing to someone other than you. I believe there are some things, albeit different things, each of you will find meaningful, and beyond—essential and critical.

DAY 2

A WINDRUNNER'S JOURNAL

I invite you to reread every sentence above which is bold and in italics. Write it down, in your own words if you wish, to remember it, reflect on it, discuss it, or even memorize it.

_____

_____

_____

_____

_____

_____

_____

_____

_____

_____

_____

_____

_____

_____

Script Writing for Act Four: The Bell Lap

At first, I was like a fly on the wall watching my patients react suddenly to facing a bear called cancer up close and personal. Then, I became a like a narrator reading a story and watching a nightmare plot unraveling in their voices and on their faces. They wanted to wake up and find it was only a dream, but they didn't. So, I became an actor joining them on stage to act out a drama none of us had rehearsed.

Now perhaps you or someone you love is on that stage, too, and you are discovering that the drama is about much more than just a disease. It is about what God wants and is waiting to do in your life which can now come into focus because of a disease. It is what I think that voice whispering to me on my Hood Canal run was talking about. Cancer changes people.

"We would rather be ruined than changed. We would rather die in our dread than climb the cross of the present and let our illusions die."

-W.H. Auden

Most of us need to be cajoled, seduced or compelled to change. Renewal is invariably preceded by some sacrifice. It is almost the only pattern in legends and literature (real life and Scripture), but we don't want to see that because we don't want to change let alone give anything up. We're about getting more, not having or controlling less – until something falls apart like getting cancer and we have no choice. The upward journey requires some unavoidable stressor. "Falling down and moving up is, in fact, the most counterintuitive message of most world religions including and most especially Christianity."[3]

Not everyone is changed in any predictable way, yet surprisingly it is often for the better. ***It was never the cancer biology that was beyond their control that made the difference. It was always something inside their control, in their hearts, minds, and decisions that did.*** For some, it came easily and they fascinated me. Clearly they knew something and had something I didn't that I wanted, because deep down inside and seldom pondered, I feared I would be in their place one day.

I had my *bears*, but they were usually only in my dreams and almost always gone I when I woke up. However, I had seen so many awful diseases and injuries, so many lives altered in their prime, so many lives cut off just when the going was getting good, that I could not escape a gnawing feeling that tragedy would befall me someday and indeed it has.

---

[3] Richard Rohr, *Falling Upward*, pg. xxii

So, I have watched, queried, and chronicled those friends and patients whose stories simply refuse to have tragic endings. Over the years, a picture has emerged and some truths have been revealed for me. I have put them to the test and they seem to be real. This book is about that picture and those truths that leap from the pages of my patients' lives. Let me show you the bread crumbs they left for us along the trail of their journeys through the dark forests of their cancers.

Science or Fiction

The scientific method taught in medical schools instructs us precisely what it takes to establish scientific fact. Research studies are performed under controlled conditions, evaluating a limited number of variables. The results are reported, reviewed, and published. However, one published paper of experimental findings does not a truth make. The methods of the experiment must also be published, the data evaluated, and then the same study must be reproduced by other reputable scientists in the same way, and must yield the same results. ***For me, it was as if my patients were doing a study with their lives and their souls. I was the scientist observing the consequences of their choices and was startled by the results.***

Now I think I understand their methods. I have passed them on to other patients, and I have tried them in my own life, and in both cases the original results have been reproduced. That is as close as I can get to the scientific method applied to the human condition, so I conclude the results are both valid and scientifically sound. When you finish reading, it will be for you to decide if it is just a bunch of hogwash or worth a try. Maybe your story is waiting to be part of a much bigger story.

For the remainder of chapter one see the full text of CANCER'S WINDRUNNERS.

Dr. Lane shares…

I have been a medical oncologist for over thirty years. Now retired, I can spend time with cancer patients in our community helping them understand what their doctors have said, what their doctors left out, and what it all means. Then I help them make decisions that respect their bodies, their families, and the life they want to lead.

Early on, I did research on how to control the side effects of cancer chemotherapy and later how to diagnose breast and prostate cancer in the least invasive way then to treat it in a boutique fashion tailored to each patient's unique cancer and circumstances. For years I worked with national cooperative cancer groups: NSABP (National Surgical Adjuvant Breast Project), SWOG (Southwest Oncology Group, and PSOC (Puget Sound Oncology Group) doing clinical research on the characterization and treatment of different cancers. I played a leadership role in conceiving, implementing, and then directing a community cancer center, Northwest Cancer Center which evolved into Puget Sound Cancer Centers, then a hospice, Northwest Hospice, and later a multidisciplinary breast center, Seattle Breast Center. That center was dedicated to saving breasts and saving lives: both biologic patient lives and their experiential quality. This was achieved through the collaborative efforts of nurses, counselors, and clergy and multiple specialty physicians—a practice unheard of then but more common today.

These responsibilities generated an opportunity to speak to patient groups, at conferences and on retreats where the focus has been on both creatively enduring the illness, but also prospering and growing through it. I continue to learn from patients and to speak when offered the opportunity.

I presently live on an island in Puget Sound, where I love taking care of the land and the beach when not sailing, climbing, or playing with one with my kids and sibs. I savor fireside reading with my wife and therapist, Suzanne (she is a Marriage and Family Therapist who practices on me regularly). Together we cherish our blended family of nine children and twenty-two grandchildren. We have started to run our own bell laps without waiting for any disease to ring our bells.

You too can make your bell lap a victory lap. For how the Windrunners were able to outrun and evade then defeat the Dragon see, *CANCER'S WINDRUNNERS*. More information on these coming books is available on my website.

***For more resources and connecting with me and
my coaching and resources, go to www.cancerdoctalk.com.***

Endnotes

1 Carteson, Laura. Professor of Psychology Stanford University. As quoted by Atul Guwande in an interview with Charlie Rose. 10/28/2014

2 Kubler-Ross, Elizabeth. *Death; the Final Stage of Growth*. NY: Simon & Schuster, 1986. p. 2.

3 Kubler-Ross, Elizabeth. *Death; the Final Stage of Growth*. NY: Simon & Schuster, 1986. "Chapter 2, Death Through Some Other Windows , Murray L. Trelease." Murray Trelease was a parish priest in the 1960s serving small Indian villages in central Alaska. He describes the customs and values in their relationship with death and dying which harkens back to their origins as nomadic tribes before the arrival of white men.

4 Ibid.

5 Scott, Stuart. ESPN News Anchor's ESPY Speech, July 17, 2014.

6 Gonzales, Laurence. *Deep Survival: Who Lives, Who Dies, and Why*. xxxxxxN.p.: ., 2004.

7 Ibid.

8 Ibid.

9 Warren, Rick. *The Purpose Driven Life*. Grand Rapids: Zondervan, 2002. p.30.

10 www.health.harvard.edu. CKANDO@FTC.GOV –attorney for the project.

11 Scott, Stuart. ESPN News Anchor's ESPY Speech, July 17, 2014

12 Lehrer, Jonah. How We Decide. Houghton Mifflin Harcourt. NY. NY. paraphrase. p. 129.

13 Ibid., p. 100.

14 Guwande MD, Atul. Harvard Professor and author of *Being Mortal: Medicine and What Matters in the End*. Interview with Charlie Rose. 10/28/2014.

15 Henly, William Ernest. *Invictus*. Paraphrased from the poem often quoted by Nelson Mandela

16 The Eagles. *Hotel California*

17 Donne, John. *No Man Is An Island*. 1629. Metaphysical poet and Dean of St Paul's Cathedral, London

18 Buechner, Frederich. *Listening to Your Life: Daily Meditationswith Frederich Buechner*. Harper Collins. 2009

19 Albom,Mitch. *Tuesdays with Morrie*. NY: Doubleday. 1997. Pg 104

20 Mauer, Kevin & Bissonnetti, Matt. *No Easy Day: The Firsthand Account of the Mission that Killed Osama Bin Laden. Dutton Penquin.* 2012.

21 Van der Post, Lauren. *A Story Like the Wind*. Harcourt Books 1972.

22 McCullough, David. *1776*. NY: Simon & Schuster, 2005.

23 http://utmost.org/destined-to-be-holy/

24 Lane, Robert F. Bell Lap Windrunners and The Dragon Vanquished. In press

25 Lewis, C.S. " Pg 42." *A Grief Observed.* NY: HarperCollins, 1989. p. 42.

26 Jobs, Steve. Stanford University Lecture, 2005

27 Kabat-Zinn, Jon. *Full Catastrophe Living: Using the Wisdom of Your Body and Mind to Face Stress, Pain and Illness.* Bantam Dell. NY, NY. 1990

28 Ballasiotes Media-Fox Island, Washington. 253 549 0015

29 Edmund Burke. Contemporary of Thomas Jefferson

30 *Gladiator,* motion picture

31 Batterson, Mark. *Wild Goose Chase XXXXX,* p. 111.

32 Buechner, Frederich. *Listening to Your Life: Daily Meditations with Frederich Buechner.* Harper Collins. 2009.

33 Weisel, Elie. *The Kingdom of Memory: Reminiscence.* Summit Books. NY. 1990. Nobel Acceptance Speech. pp. 235-36

34 Credence Clearwater Revival. *Someday Never Comes*

35 XXXXXX *The Etiquette of Illness: What to Say When You Can't Find the Words.* Bloomsbury USA. 2004.

36 *Being Mortal: Medicine and What Matters in the End.*

37 Cristakis, Michael. *New England Journal of Medicine. 357;4.* July 26, 2007

38 Ibid.

39 Wright, AA et al. *Journal of the American Medical Association* 300:1665-1673. 2008

CPSIA information can be obtained
at www.ICGtesting.com
Printed in the USA
BVHW051225290323
661369BV00004B/125